BIOKINETIC EXERCISES

A Guide to Realigning Your Body Naturally

Wayne Topping, Ph.D., L.M.T.

Published by:
Topping International Institute, Inc.
2505 Cedarwood Ave, Suite 3
Bellingham, WA, 98225 U.S.A
Phone: (360) 647-2703 Fax: (360) 647-0164
www.wellnesskinesiology.com

Special Note:

The procedures and techniques described in this manual are solely for information and/or research purposes. The author and Topping International Institute, Inc. are not dispensing medical advice, diagnoses, or prescriptions, either directly or indirectly for any reader or student. We make no recommendations or representations concerning the physiological effects for any of these procedures or ideas reported. This information is not intended to offer medical, physiological or other professional services, and whenever persons find themselves in need of treatment by a medical professional, we encourage them to see a duly licensed medical practitioner. Persons using the challenges, tests, corrections or recommendations reported here, do so entirely at their own risk.

ISBN 0-935299-13-0

1st Published   1999
2nd Printing   2006

Copyright© 1998 by Topping International Institute, Inc. Artwork© D.W. Miller 1996

All rights reserved. No part of this book may be reproduced, stored, or transmitted in any form or by any means, including electronic, mechanical, or photocopying without the prior written permission of the publisher or the author.

Credits:
Photography: Rich Dryden
Models: Kathryn Wenona Zahlis, Eric Ward
Art: D.W. Miller
Layout Concept: Norbert Alvermann
Layout & Cover Design: Cathrine Levan

Printed in the United States by:
McNaughton & Gunn, Inc.
960 Woodland Drive
Saline, MI 48176 U.S.A

Acknowledgments:

Since Dr. George Goodheart introduced Applied Kinesiology in the early 1960's and Dr. John Thie introduced Touch for Health in the 1970's there has been rapid development of many schools of kinesiology. Within this very fertile and dynamic field many techniques and methodologies have been shared and borrowed as practitioners and trainers are continually upgrading, simplifying and extending their kinesiological applications.

I especially thank Dr. John Thie for his development of Touch for Health and for his vision which has helped establish it in at least 55 countries. I am very grateful to John and his wife Carrie for their friendship over the years. Touch for Health was my first introduction to kinesiology back in 1976.

However, much of my early kinesiological training was in the field of Biokinesiology developed beginning in the early 1970's by John and Margaret Barton. I took three month's training with John in 1980 to become a biokinesiology instructor and have taught it extensively in many parts of the world. I have really appreciated my friendship with John and Margaret and valued their willingness to share experiences and answer questions. Because of the vast amount of valuable information within Biokinesiology I have chosen as one of my roles over the years to present at conferences various biokinesiological procedures which can easily be integrated into other kinesiologies to increase the choices available to each practitioner. One of these methods is working with Biokinetic Exercises. Originally the Bartons (the Biokinesiology Institute) presented about 180 of these passive exercises in their book *Be Your Own Chiropractor* (1979) arranged according to the 20 acupuncture meridians.

Increasingly over the years as Touch for Health has led to the development by Dr. Bruce and Joan Dewe of the Professional Kinesiology Practitioner series it has been obvious that there is need for a book presenting biokinetic exercises for people familiar with Touch for Health and the Professional Kinesiology Practitioner workshop series. In this book I have included biokinetic exercises for the muscles, tendons and ligaments we work with in Touch for Health I, II, III, & IV, Professional Kinesiology Practitioner I, and the eight extra meridians (my book, *Balancing the Bodies Energies*).

There is very little original research on my part in this book. The muscle tests are drawn from Touch for Health, the Professional Kinesiology Practitioner series, and Biokinesiology. Most of the information on how to circuit localize the tissue, and the biokinetic exercises come from Biokinesiology. I have reorganized this material for a specific audience, those using one of the many forms of kinesiology.

I am very grateful to John Barton for his permission to use the biokinetic exercises developed as part of Biokinesiology and for his many helpful suggestions as I was putting this text together. Many heartfelt thanks to Risteard de Barra and Dr. Clyde Ford, D.C. for their critical reading of the text and their many helpful suggestions. Also my European Wellness Kinesiology™ Instructors for advice including Christos Cavadias, Dominique Plovier and Marc Willems for their written comments.

Many thanks to Rich Dryden for your wonderful photographs and to Kathryn Wenona Zahlis and Eric Ward for the many hours posing for those photographs. A big thank you to David Miller for your excellent artwork.

Finally, many thanks to Sandy Bonnickson, Finnian Byrnes and Cathrine Levan for the countless hours required to transform my handwritten notes into a text that is esthetically far more appealing and readable.

-Wayne W. Topping

Table of Contents:

PART I

INTRODUCTION TO BIOKINETIC EXERCISES
What Are Biokinetic Exercises?...9
How Do Biokinetic Exercises Work?..10
How Long Do We Hold the Biokinetic Position?..10
How to Know Whether You Have the Optimum Position...11
Biokinetic Exercises for the Low Back 12
Biokinetic Exercises for the Neck and Shoulders...14

USING MUSCLE MONITORING
Circuit Localizing...16
Circuit Localizing Different Types of Tissues..16
Circuit Localizing to Find the Optimum Position..17
Circuit Localizing to Determine How Long to Hold the Biokinetic Position...........18

HOW TO USE BIOKINETIC EXERCISES
How to Use Biokinetic Exercises..19
How to Use this Book..19

PART II

TISSUES AND CORRECTIONS
Abductor Hallucis...22
Adductor Brevis..23
Adductor Longus..24
Adductor Magnus...25
Adductor Pollicis..26
Biceps Brachii...27
Biceps Femoris...28
Brachioradialis..29
Buccinator...30
Coracobrachialis...31
Deltoid Anterior...32
Deltoid Middle..33
Deltoid Posterior..34
Diaphragm...35
Dorsal Interossei..36
Extensor Carpi Radialis Longus..37
Extensor Carpi Ulnaris..38

Table of Contents:

Extensor Digitorum Brevis...39
Extensor Digitorum Longus...40
Extensor Hallucis Brevis...41
Extensor Hallucis Longus...42
Extensor Pollicis Longus...43
External Oblique...44
Flexor Carpi Radialis...45
Flexor Carpi Ulnaris...46
Flexor Digitorum Brevis...47
Flexor Digitorum Longus...48
Flexor Digitorum Profundus...49
Flexor Digitorum Superficialis (sublimis)...50
Flexor Hallucis Brevis...51
Flexor Hallucis Longus...52
Flexor Pollicis Brevis...53
Flexor Pollicis Longus...54
Gastrocnemius...55
Gluteus Maximus...56
Gluteus Medius...57
Gluteus Minimus...58
Gracilis...59
Iliacus...60
Infraspinatus...61
Internal Oblique...62
Latissimus Dorsi...63
Levator Scapulae...64
Lumbricals (of the foot)...65
Lumbricals (of the hand)...66
Masseter...67
Obliquus Capitis Inferior...68
Obliquus Capitis Superior...69
Opponens Digiti Minimi...70
Opponens Pollicis...71
Palmaris Longus...72
Pectineus...73
Pectoralis Major Clavicular...74
Pectoralis Major Sternal...75
Pectoralis Minor...76
Peroneus Tertius...77
Piriformis...78
Plantar Interossei...79
Popliteus...80

Table of Contents:

Pronator Quadratus..81
Pronator Teres...82
Psoas Major..83
Pterygoid Lateral (External Pteryoid)...................................84
Pterygoid Medial (Internal Pteryoid)....................................85
Pyramidalis..86
Quadratus Lumborum...87
Rectus Abdominis..88
Rectus Capitis Anterior...89
Rectus Capitis Lateralis..90
Rectus Capitis Posterior Major 91
Rectus Capitis Posterior Minor 92
Rectus Femoris (1 of 4 parts of Quadriceps)......................93
Rhomboid Major...94
Rhomboid Minor...95
Rotatores Brevis..96
Rotatores Longus..97
Sartorius..98
Semimembranosus..99
Semitendinosus...100
Serratus Anterior...101
Serratus Anterior #5 (tendon)..102
Shoulder Capsular Ligament Anterior.................................103
Soleus..104
Sternocleidomastoid..105
Subclavius..106
Subscapularis...107
Supinator..108
Supraspinatus..109
Temporalis..110
Tensor Fasciae Latae..111
Teres Major...112
Teres Minor...113
Tibialis Anterior..114
Tibialis Posterior..115
Transversus Abdominis 116
Trapezius (lower division)..117
Trapezius (middle division)..118
Trapezius (upper division)...119
Triceps Brachii...120
Vastus Intermedius (1 of 4 parts of Quadriceps)..............121
Vastus Lateralis (1 of 4 parts of Quadriceps)...................122
Vastus Medialis (1 of 4 parts of Quadriceps)....................123

Table of Contents:

PART III

APPENDIX A: GLOSSARY OF TERMS
Directional Terms...125
Terms of Movement..125
Miscellaneous Anatomical Terms...126

APPENDIX B: MUSCLE MONITORING REVIEW
Review of Procedures...128
What is Muscle Monitoring?..128
    Deltoid...128
    Anterior Deltoid..129
    Techniques to Balance the Deltoid Muscle...129
    Techniques to Balance the Anterior Deltoid Muscle.............................129
Testing for a 'Balanced Indicator Muscle'...130
Pre-checks and Corrections for Accurate Indicator Muscle Biofeedback........130
    Hydration: The Hair Tug Test...130
    Switching..130
    Switching: A Verbal Test..131
    Electromagnetic Screening Test..131
    Over Energy..132
    Auriculars...133
    Eye Directions..133

REFERENCES...134

INDEX...135

Part I

Introduction to Biokinetic Exercises
Using Muscle Monitoring
How to Use Biokinetic Exercises

Introduction to Biokinetic Exercises

What Are Biokinetic Exercises?

In Biokinesiology we take a wholistic approach to balancing the body, believing that if we use emotional, nutritional and physical approaches simultaneously we bring the body into balance more quickly and it is likely to be a more lasting balance. One of the physical methods we use to restore balance is the biokinetic exercise.

Biokinetic exercises are passive exercises that use position-releasing to balance kinetic tissues (muscles, tendons, etc.) that are either too weak (hypotonic) or too tense (hypertonic).

The aim of each exercise is to shorten the distance between the origin and the insertion of the muscle, tendon, ligament or fascia. If the person simply contracts the tissue and holds that position, it won't go back into balance. However, if external pressure or gravity is used to maintain the same shortened position, the tissue can relax fully and go back into balance. The therapist or practitioner can sometimes assist the client or patient by holding them in the desired position - particularly if they are very young or elderly. However, one of the features that is very attractive about biokinetic exercises is that clients can do it for themselves. I'm sure that the more clients can do for themselves, the more they take self-responsibility, the more likely they are to get the positive health-enhancing results they are after.

John and Margaret Barton, the founders of Biokinesiology developed biokinetic exercises during the 1970's and published a book *Be Your Own Chiropractor Through Biokinetic Exercises* in 1979, where they described and illustrated approximately 180 of these passive exercises. Most of the hundreds of tissues described in the *Atlas*, another publication from the Biokinesiology Institute, are accompanied by written descriptions of their biokinetic exercises.

While biokinetic exercises are well known among biokinesiologists they are far less known among other kinesiologists. This book's major objective is to introduce these valuable exercises to the broader kinesiological community. With this in mind I have taken all the muscles worked with in Touch for Health I, II, III, & IV, Professional Kinesiology Practitioner I, and the Eight Extra Meridian work and placed them in alphabetical order for ease of access.

First we will look at the underlying principles. Then we will show how the biokinetic exercise procedure can be applied to specific areas of the body – the neck and shoulders, and the low back. This can be done without muscle testing, using "noticing" as feedback to let us know how successful the biokinetic exercise has been.

How do we know which biokinetic exercise to use? Identifying the specific tissue that is out of balance allows us to turn to that muscle or tendon in the book, view a photograph and read a verbal description of the biokinetic exercise. The tissue that is out of balance can be identified through manual muscle testing, as we've been doing in Touch for Health and related kinesiologies, or more accurately through circuit localizing. The advantage of circuit localizing is that we can define the type of tissue involved – whether it is muscle, tendon, ligament, or fascia. This is useful information because the biokinetic position is held for different lengths of time depending upon the type of tissue that is out of balance.

These biokinetic exercises are relatively simple to use, to teach to your clients, and they can be integrated well with other kinesiological corrections. For example, if you find that your client has chronic low back pain and the psoas major muscle shows up as the top priority correction, then, as part of the client's growth work you could assign them the biokinetic exercise for the psoas major muscle the first thing in the morning and the last thing at night (or at whatever times muscle testing indicates would be most appropriate).

Introduction to Biokinetic Exercises

How Do Biokinetic Exercises Work?

If you saw a person with their palm on their forehead and their elbow resting on a table to prop their head up, very likely you would recognize that the person is stressed. Ask them why they have their palm on their forehead and they probably couldn't tell you. The point is, it probably was not a conscious choice. However, kinesiologists would recognize that they are doing something reflexly or innately (emotional stress release) that is having a balancing effect on their mind/body. If you observe people, you will recognize that we often do things reflexly or innately that have survival value.

When you burn your hand your first reflex action is to pull your hand in towards you - not further away from you, or to the side - but towards you. Whenever a muscle gets injured the reflex action is to contract, to pull the injured part closer to you. With the biokinetic exercise that is what we are doing, putting tissues into their contracted positions. Another example. Take one of your clients who has a chronic psoas muscle imbalance or low back pain. Ask them how they sleep and the chances are very high that it will be in the fetal position. Why? Because it "feels more comfortable". Moreover, if they slept in any other position they would probably experience more low back pain. With the psoas muscle out of balance the following structural symptoms can be experienced. Difficulty in standing upright. Low back ache. Lower back malalignment. Hip pains. Desire to curl up when in bed. By sleeping in the fetal position, on the side with one or both knees pulled up toward the chest, the person is, in effect, doing a biokinetic exercise. They don't know how it works. They just know that it is more comfortable if they sleep this way.

We know empirically that biokinetic exercises work. We know that people sometimes do them unconsciously. But we don't know precisely how they work. When you injure a muscle the reflex, protective response is to pull in closer to the core of the body to nurse the injured part. Holding the muscle in its shortened state causes it to relax. It may be that the brain can then allow this more relaxed pain free state to be transferred back into the extended state.

Dr. George Goodheart has shown that most pain is due to weakness in the opposing muscles. Clients will often describe pain where muscles are hypertonic or too tight. However, if the opposing muscles are palpated they will usually elicit pain. They are sore because they are weak or hypotonic. Whether muscles are painful (hypertonic) or sore (hypotonic) they are out of balance. Holding such muscles in a shortened relaxed state (not simply contracted) may allow the proprioceptors such as spindle cells to cause the brain to change the tone of the muscle.

How Long Do We Hold the Biokinetic Position?

Biokinesiology research has shown that different types of tissues require different lengths of time to get back into balance. As a general rule of thumb, minimum times are:

> Thirty seconds for muscles
> One minute for tendons
> Two minutes for ligaments
> Five minutes for fascias

Later we will show you how to use muscle testing to determine specifically what type of tissue is out of balance and therefore the amount of time required to hold the biokinetic position. In the meantime you may want to hold each position for about a minute if you don't know whether your imbalanced tissue is a muscle or tendon (which is the problem most of the time). If some of the discomfort remains you could hold the position longer as you may be dealing with a ligament or fascia.

Introduction to Biokinetic Exercises

How to Know Whether You Have the Optimum Position

NOTES:

In the correct position the imbalanced tissue should be free of pain or the pain should be greatly minimized. Hold the arm, leg or head in the position that brings the ends of the imbalanced tissue as close together as possible. Assess what it feels like. If the pain is gone, that is the correct position to hold. If some pain is still noticeable, change the positioning slightly looking for the position where the pain disappears or is at its least. Then do the same correction for the other side of the body.

Remember to move into and out of each position slowly. When tissues are brought back into proper tone they can cause bones to change their positions relative to each other. For this reason, move SLOWLY into and out of each position.

Don't hold a biokinetic position if it causes increased pain. Attempt the same position on the other side of the body. If this doesn't cause pain, hold this position first. Then it may be that the first position can be done without pain.

If in doubt about holding a particular position, it is better to err on the cautious side and not do it. If you are assisting a client or friend with biokinetic exercises, remember to inform them that they are responsible for giving you feedback as to whether the pain is gone, less, the same, or more as you attempt to find the optimal position. Go slowly. You need to be careful working with any part of the body that is already in pain.

Introduction to Biokinetic Exercises

Biokinetic Exercises for the Low Back

To illustrate how biokinetic exercises can be used to relieve pain in the body we will focus specifically on the low back region. The general procedure is presented first, then exercises for three of the major muscles in the low back region – serratus posterior inferior, quadratus lumborum, and multifidus spinea superficial – as first presented in *Creative Health*, Vol. 5(6), 1981.

General Procedure

1. Find the sore muscle by pressing into the tender area.

2. SLOWLY, GENTLY twist and bend the body around until you find the exact position that seems to make the sore muscle relax. You will notice this by just poking into the sore area and moving the body slightly, then poke again. When you have found the position that allows the best contraction of that muscle, it will simply relax; the tenderness will be greatly reduced.

3. You hold, for 30 to 60 seconds, the exact position that makes the sore muscle relax.

4. You VERY SLOWLY straighten up and then do the same exercise on the opposite side of the body. REMEMBER TO MOVE SLOWLY!

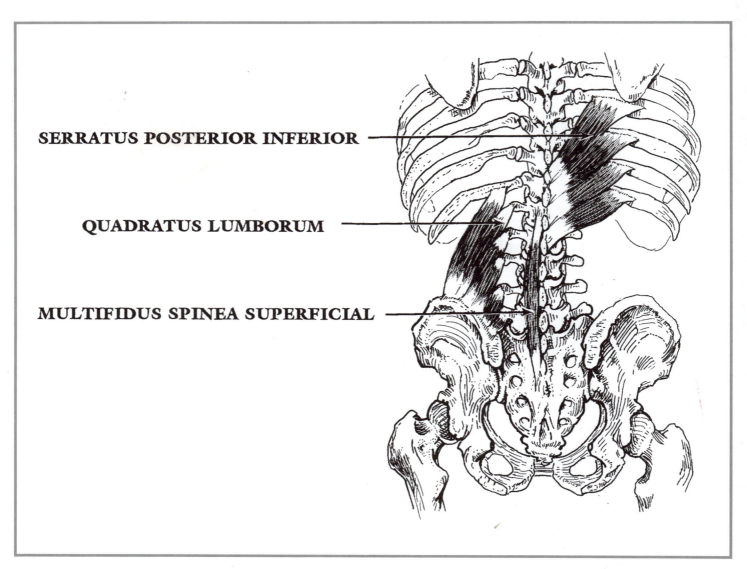

Introduction to Biokinetic Exercises

EXAMPLE 1:
This is for muscles that go from your spine up to your lower ribs (**serratus posterior inferior**).

1. Slowly twist your upper body far to the right.

2. Press your right hip up and forward with your right hand.

3. Arch back and tilt to the right.

4. Hold this position for 30 seconds; then straighten up slowly. Repeat the same position on the left side.

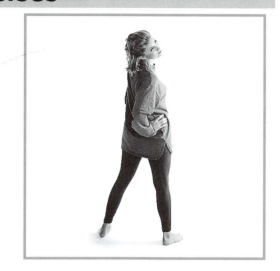

EXAMPLE 2:
This exercise is for the muscles that go between the lowest rib and low spine down to the hip bone (**quadratus lumborum**).

1. Arch back slightly.

2. Bend to the right side about 30 to 45 degrees.

3. Put your right hand on your right hip and press it upwards.

4. Hold this position for 30 seconds; then straighten up slowly. Repeat the same relaxing position on the left side.

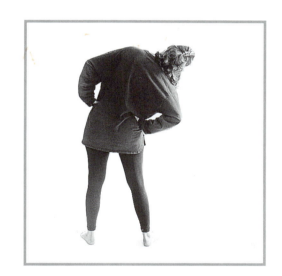

EXAMPLE 3:
This exercise is for the muscles that go directly up the back very close to the spine (**multifidus spinea superficial**).

1. GENTLY, CAREFULLY arch back until the muscle feels relaxed.

2. Hold this position for 30 seconds, then straighten up VERY-VERY SLOWLY! If need be, lean against a wall for support.

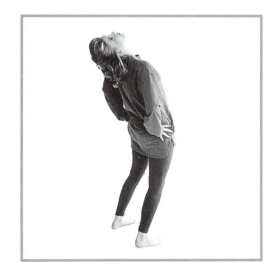

Introduction to Biokinetic Exercises

Biokinetic Exercises for the Neck and Shoulders

There are many muscles in the neck and shoulder areas. However, to illustrate the procedures we will describe just three - **upper trapezius** (trapezius, upper division), **levator scapulae**, and **sternocleidomastoid** (anterior neck flexors). The general procedure is the same as for the low back and is repeated below.

General Procedure

1. Find the sore muscle by pressing into the tender area.

2. SLOWLY, GENTLY twist the body around until you find the exact position that seems to make the sore muscle relax. You will notice this by just poking into the sore area and moving the body slightly, then poke again. When you have found the position that causes the best contraction of that muscle, it will simply relax; the tenderness will be greatly reduced.

3. You hold, for 30 to 60 seconds, the exact position that makes the sore muscle relax.

4. You VERY SLOWLY straighten up. Then do the same exercise on the opposite side of the body. REMEMBER TO MOVE SLOWLY!

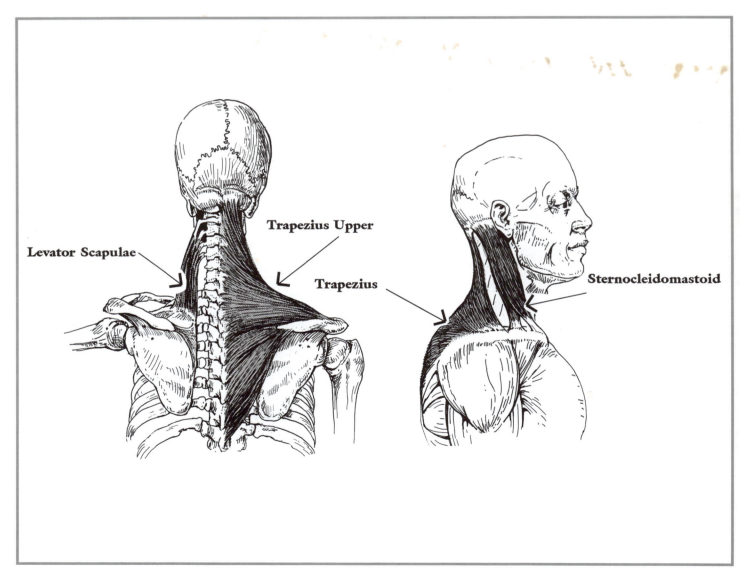

Introduction to Biokinetic Exercises

EXAMPLE 1:
This exercise is to balance the very shoulder muscles where most of us accumulate our work-related tension (**upper trapezius muscles**).

1. Place your left palm on your back between your shoulder blades by reaching up over your left shoulder. Keep the elbow high in the air.

2. Grasp the left elbow with your right hand by reaching behind the head.

3. Turn your face 20° to the right, and tilt your head 45° to the left. Arch back and hold this position for 30 seconds.

4. Repeat the same position on the right side.

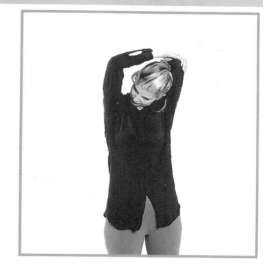

EXAMPLE 2:
This exercise is for muscles in the back of the shoulder and neck which are often found weak (causing the neck to twist with the head staying level) and are often a source of pain (**levator scapulae muscles**).

1. Sit on the floor with your legs comfortably in front of you, placing your hands together behind you with your fingers pointing back.

2. Lean and arch back, facing up to the ceiling.

3. Tilt your head 45 degrees to the left and hold this position for 30 seconds. Repeat the same position on the right side.

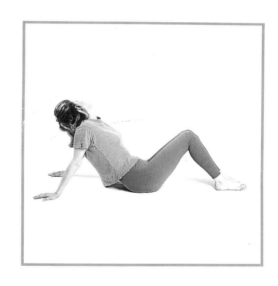

EXAMPLE 3:
This exercise is to balance muscles on the front and sides of the neck that are often weak and a source of headaches and shoulder tension (**sternocleidomastoid muscles**).

1. With back straight, turn head 10° to the right.

2. Tilt your head down forward and tuck the chin in.

3. Gently push down on top of your head and hold this position for 30 seconds.

4. Repeat the same position on the right side.

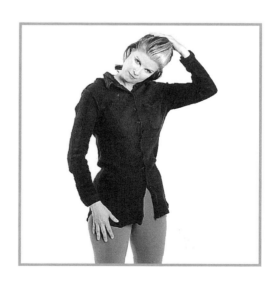

Using Muscle Monitoring

Circuit Localizing

Principle

The deltoid muscle or deltoid anterior muscle can be used as an indicator muscle while the client or practitioner circuit localizes or touches the fingertips to various body tissues. The indicator muscle is thus used as a biofeedback instrument to detect electrical imbalances within the body.

Method

1. Identify a functional Indicator Muscle (I.M.), i.e., check for dehydration, switching, central meridian overenergy, auriculars, eye directions, and make any corrections needed. Check in contraction, then in extension (the antagonists). Use spindle cells to sedate then tonify the I.M.

2. Client or practitioner touches the finger tips directly into a specific tissue while practitioner tests the I.M. Either:

3. (a) Indicator muscle (I.M.) switches off: tissue is out of balance, i.e., **"weak"** in biokinesiology terminology;
    or
   (b) I.M. remains switched on. Practitioner runs hand up center of client's body (central meridian) while continuing to circuit localize the tissue, then tests I.M.

      (i) I.M. remains switched on: tissue is **in balance**.

      (ii) I.M. switches off: in biokinesiological terms we say the tissue is **"overstressed"**.

Circuit Localizing Different Types of Tissues

Principle

Circuit localizing allows us to identify the type of tissue that is out of balance. This lets us know how long to hold the biokinetic exercise position.

Method

The nerve endings under the fingernails are our most sensitive detecting units. Our objective, therefore, is to have the undersurface of the fingernails in contact with as much of the tissue we are investigating as possible. Below we have tips for various types of tissues.

Surface Muscles: Grasp the muscle with the fingers pointing directly into it.

Deep Muscles: Press fingertips deeply into the belly of the muscle.

Fascia: Angle tips of thumb and fingers so that the undersurface of fingernails cut across fascial surface at depth.

Tendons: Press fingertips into area where muscle attaches into bone. Say audibly to testee "You feel adequate" while circuit localizing a tendon or ligament and the unlocked I.M. should lock. "You feel inadequate" should unlock the I.M. again. This is a way to differentiate between muscles and tendons or ligaments.

Ligaments: Press fingertips into area between bones. The I.M. should lock when you say "you feel adequate", and it should unlock when you say "you feel inadequate". This is a way to distinguish between ligaments or tendons, and muscles.

Using Muscle Monitoring

Circuit Localizing to Find the Optimum Position

If you are working with a client or friend, circuit localizing the tissue while he or she is in the proposed position will let you know if the position is optimal or could be improved.

To understand how this is possible, we need some background on the three main conditions of a tissue that are identified in Biokinesiology.

(A) The tissue can be **weak**, i.e., when we circuit localize it and test an indicator muscle (I.M.) the I.M. unlocks.

(B) It can be **overstressed** or have too much energy. In this case the I.M. will not unlock while circuit localizing the tissue. However, the I.M. will unlock when either the practitioner, or the client, runs a hand up the central meridian on the client from groin to chin to surge some additional energy through the circuit involving that tissue.

(C) It can be in balance or **strong**. Here the indicator muscle is locked when the tissue is circuit localized, and it remains strong or locked after a hand is passed up the client's central meridian.

Each tissue has an antagonist tissue and their relationship can be exemplified by considering a seesaw. There are three possible conditions.

(i) Tissue A and its antagonist tissue, B, are both in balance (strong).

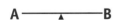

(ii) When tissue A is weak the antagonist tissue, B, will be overstressed.

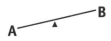

(iii) When tissue A becomes overstressed, then the antagonist tissue B becomes weak.

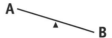

(iv) If tissue A is weak, the optimal biokinetic exercise will temporarily allow it to circuit localize (CL) as being overstressed. If it CLs as strong, the position is close but not ideal. If the tissue CLs as weak, the biokinetic exercise position is ineffective.

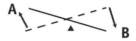

If tissue A is originally overstressed, the optimum biokinetic exercise position will temporarily cause the tissue to CL as weak. A biokinetic exercise position that is close will cause the tissue to CL as strong. When the position is ineffective it will still CL as overstressed, i.e., no change.

To summarize, if we have a muscle, tendon, ligament or fascia that circuit localized as **WEAK** or **OVERSTRESSED** we have the following possibilities:

Muscle, Tendon, Ligament, Or Fascia is Originally	Biokinetic Exercise Position Causes Tissue To Circuit Localize As:	Biokinetic Exercise Position Is:
Weak	Weak	Not Effective
Weak	Strong	Close
Weak	Overstressed	Optimum
Overstressed	Overstressed	Not Effective
Overstressed	Strong	Close
Overstressed	Weak	Optimum

Using Muscle Monitoring

Circuit Localizing to Determine How Long to Hold the Biokinetic Position

Situation: The muscle you are testing unlocks.

Question: How long do we need to hold the biokinetic position to balance this muscle?

Let us take the **rhomboid major** muscle (page 94) as an example.

1. Muscle test the rhomboid major on left side, then right side of the body. Let's say it unlocks on the left.

2. Practitioner touches the finger tips into the left rhomboid major **muscle** midway between the thoracic spine (2nd-5th thoracic vertebrae) and the medial border of the scapula. Say "love, love" out loud then retest the muscle.

    (a) If the muscle now **locks**, it is the **muscle** that needs to be balanced and the biokinetic exercise needs to be held for at least 30 seconds.

    (b) If the muscle still **unlocks**, it is not the muscle that is out of balance. Go to step 3.

3. Practitioner touches the fingertips into the **tendon** for the left rhomboid major, immediately to the left of the spine alongside the second to fifth thoracic vertebrae and says "love, love" out loud.

    (a) If the muscle test now **locks**, it is the **tendon** that needs to be balanced and the biokinetic exercise needs to be held for at least one minute.

    (b) If the muscle still **unlocks**, it is not the tendon that is out of balance. Go to step 4.

4. Practitioner flexes fingers and thumb so as to localize the **fascia** overlying the left rhomboid major muscle and says "love, love" out loud.

    (a) If the muscle now **locks**, it is the **fascia** that needs to be balanced and the biokinetic exercise needs to be held for five minutes.

    (b) If the muscle still **unlocks**, it is probably not the rhomboid major muscle, tendon or fascia that is out of balance. Client could do the rhomboid major biokinetic exercise to see if it changes the muscle test, or look for some other imbalanced tissue that is causing that muscle test to unlock.

How to Use Biokinetic Exercises

How To Use Biokinetic Exercises

1. Find a sore muscle and attempt to find a position of contraction that will release the tension. Hold. See *Biokinetic Exercises for the Low Back*, pp.11-12, or *Biokinetic Exercises for the Neck and Shoulders*, pp 13-14.

2. If you know the name of the weak or over-stressed tissue, locate it in the table of contents at the front of this book. Turn to the relevant page and read off a description for that particular biokinetic exercise.

3. If you cannot name the a particular tissue that is sore of painful, identify a muscle that appears to be in a similar position. Locate that muscle in the table of contents, then turn to that muscle description because the described biokinetic exercise may be close enough to be effective for you particular imbalance.

4. Remember that in Touch for Health and kinesiology generally, we test a muscle in its contracted position. With a biokinetic exercise our objective is to duplicate the positioning, or to take the muscle further into contraction without actively using it.

5. Circuit localize the tissue to determine whether it is weak or overstressed. Bring the origin and insertion as close together as possible. Then circuit localize the tissue again to see if it is now opposite its previous condition. If not, keep repositioning until you have the desired state. Hold.

How to Use This Book

On pages 22-123 we have muscles, tendons, and ligaments taken from Touch for Health I-IV; Professional Kinesiology Practitioner I; and our Eight Extra Meridians work. They are arranged in alphabetical order for ease of access. Where a muscle such as deltoid is commonly divided into three different portions, they are ordered sequentially deltoid anterior, deltoid middle, and deltoid posterior, rather than as anterior deltoid, middle deltoid, and posterior deltoid and showing up in quite separate areas of the book. This applies to the tibialis, trapezius muscles, etc. However, the individual portions of the abdominals, hamstrings, and quadriceps are sufficiently well recognized that they are listed alphabetically. I have followed standard international and anglo-saxon terminology with the exception that I use names such as deltoid and rhomboid rather than the less commonly used names deltoideus and rhomboideus. Alternative names are listed in the index. For example, just among kinesiology reference texts that I use, external oblique is also named external oblique abdominal, external abdominal oblique, abdominal oblique external, and obliquus externus abdominis. Here I have elected to use the name most commonly used in America today.

Origins and **insertions** are given in more detail than in Touch for Health for those who wish to circuit localize the tendons with accuracy. Two **methods of testing** are described. All kinesiologists are familiar with **muscle testing** to clearly indicate that we are not interested in testing the crude strength of the muscle. In Biokinesiology **circuit localizing** (called therapy localizing in Biokinesiology literature) is our major means of testing for tissue imbalances. If the indicator muscle unlocks, you should be able to circuit localize the specific tissue that is out of balance. Say "love" while continuing to localize the tissue, then remove your fingertips and check to see if

How to Use Biokinetic Exercises

the previously unlocked muscle is now switched on. If so, you've correctly identified the tissue that is out of balance. Where and how you circuit localize should tell you what type of tissue you are dealing with. The biokinetic exercises are the same for muscles, tendons and fascia. Hold for 30 seconds, one minute or five minutes depending upon the type of tissue that you identified.

Some of the muscles, e.g. rectus capitis lateralis, are sufficiently small that they cannot be muscle tested directly. A **surrogate muscle** can be used as in the Professional Kinesiology Practitioner program and in Edu-Kinesthetics. However, circuit localizing can be used to differentiate between rectus capitis lateralis and the rectus capitis posterior muscles. Circuit localizing can also let you know when you have the optimum biokinetic positions.

Throughout the text we strove for a balance between scientific accuracy and simple terminology while aiming for variety. We may not have always succeeded. If you can see any corrections that are needed, please contact the publisher.

Movement terminology and miscellaneous anatomical terms used throughout the text are listed on pages 125-127 in the Appendix.

NOTES:

Part II

Tissues and Corrections

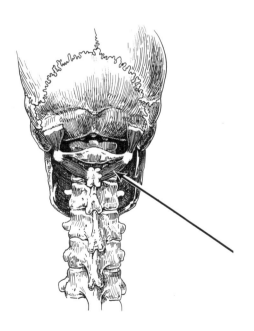
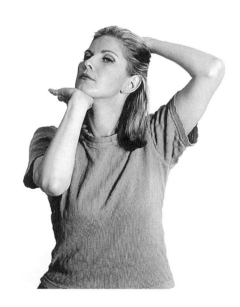

Abductor Hallucis

abductor = moves part away from midline; hallucis = of the great toe

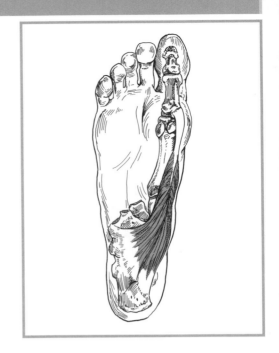

Muscle Facts

Origin:
Plantar surface of the medial process of the tuberosity of the calcaneus and adjacent ligament.

Insertion:
With the medial tendon of the flexor hallucis brevis into the medial side of the base of the proximal phalanx of the great toe.

Action:
Abducts the great toe from the midline of the foot.

Method of Testing

Muscle Test:
With the great toe in abduction (separated from second toe), pressure is on the medial side of the toe to move it towards the second toe.

Circuit Localize:
Medial margin plantar surface of foot midway between heel and proximal end of great toe.

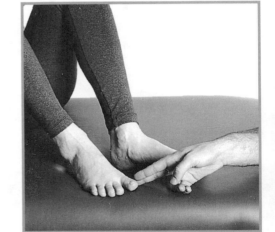

Biokinetic Exercise

1. Grasp your left great toe and pull it out to the right, twisting it to the right.
2. Press it toward the inside of your heel, pulling the inside of your heel forward at the same time. Keep the great toe straight.

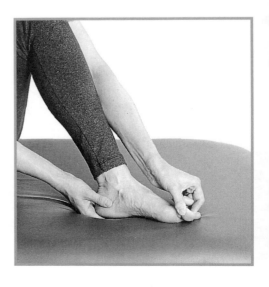

Adductor Brevis

adductor = moves part closer to midline; brevis = short

Muscle Facts

Origin:
Outer surface of inferior ramus of pubis.

Insertion:
The upper half of the linea aspera.

Action:
Adduction of thigh at the hip. Assists in thigh flexion and medial rotation at the hip.

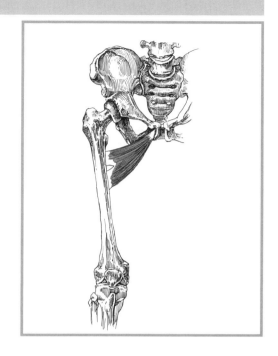

Method of Testing

Muscle Test:
Client supine, legs together and toes up. Pull one leg out laterally while stabilizing the opposite leg.

Circuit Localize:
Two thumb widths below top of inner thigh, medial aspect.

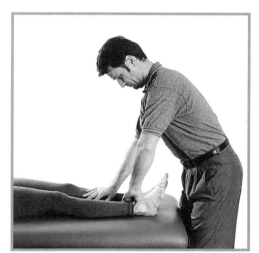

Biokinetic Exercise

Lying on your back, bring your left knee up towards your right shoulder. Grasp behind left thigh and pull it toward your abdomen. Rest.

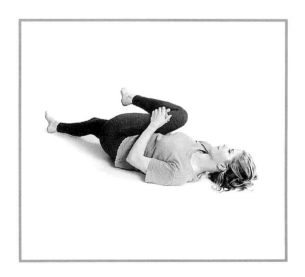

Adductor Longus

adductor = moves part closer to midline; longus = long

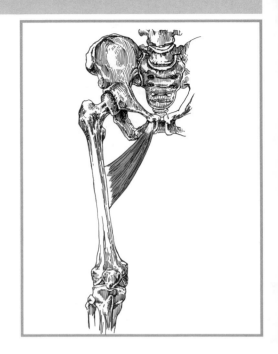

Muscle Facts

Origin:
Pubic crest and symphysis pubis.

Insertion:
The linea aspera in the middle third of the thigh.

Action:
Adduction of thigh at the hip joint. Assists in thigh flexion, medial rotation at the hip.

Method of Testing

Muscle Test:
Client supine, legs extended, toes turned out. Pull one leg out laterally while stabilizing the opposite leg.

Circuit Localize:
In line between the pubic bone and the anterior medial part of the middle part of the thigh.

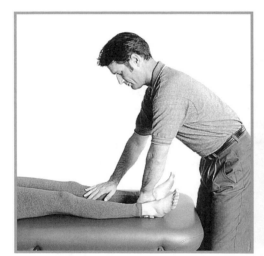

Biokinetic Exercise

1. Stand up and place your left foot on the right side of your right foot, keeping your legs straight and your feet pointing forwards.
2. Bend forwards and to the left from the hips, keep your upper torso straight. Rest.
3. It is often helpful to grasp the outside back of the left knee and pull it towards the right hip.

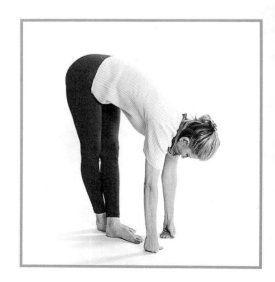

Adductor Magnus

adductor = moves part closer to midline; magnus = large

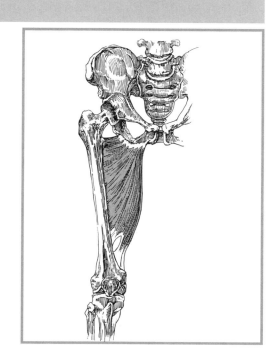

Muscle Facts
Origin:
Posterior Fibers (Long Head of Biokinesiology): Ischial tuberosity.
Anterior Fibers (Short Head of Biokinesiology): Ramus of ischium and inferior ramus of the pubis.

Insertion:
Broad aponeurosis into whole length of linea aspera and the medial supracondylar line. Tendon into adductor tubercle on medial condyle of femur.

Action:
The whole muscle adducts the thigh at the hip joint. The upper (anterior) fibers assist with inward rotation and flexion of the thigh; the lower (posterior) fibers assist with inward rotation and extension of the thigh.

Method of Testing
Muscle Test: Posterior Fibers: Client supine. Raise leg 6" from table. Rotate foot in 30°. Pressure is against medial ankle to push it outwards.
Anterior Fibers: Client supine. Raise leg 6" from table. Foot neutral. Pressure is against medial ankle to push it outwards.

Circuit Localize:
Posterior Fibers: One palm below groin, on medial aspect of thigh, pressing in very deeply.
Anterior Fibers: One palm below groin, 4 finger widths anterior of the median line on the thigh, pressing in very deeply.

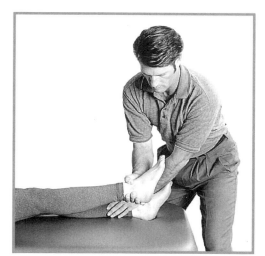

Biokinetic Exercise
1. Stand with your feet two feet apart.
2. Turn your feet out 60° and bend towards the outside of your left foot.
3. Keeping your upper torso straight, bend at the hips.

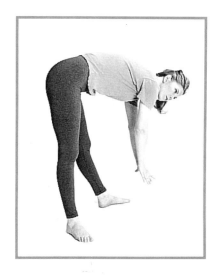

Adductor Pollicis

adductor = moves part closer to midline; pollicis = of the thumb

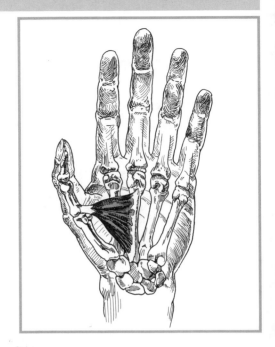

Muscle Facts
Origin:
Oblique Head: Capitate bone, bases of the second and third metacarpals, and the intercarpal ligaments.
Transverse Head: Distal two-thirds of the palmar surface of the third metacarpal bone.

Insertion:
The two heads converge to insert on the ulnar side of the base of the proximal phalanx of the thumb.

Action:
Adduction of the thumb at the carpometacarpal joint. Adduction and assists in flexion of the thumb at the metacarpophalangeal joint.

Method of Testing
Muscle Test:
Stabilize the hand, especially the center of the palm. The thumb is held close to the palm. Pressure is against the distal end of the proximal phalanx of the thumb to move it away from the palm.

Circuit Localize:
Oblique Head: Midway along fleshy pad of thumb, closer to palm.
Transverse Head: Midway between second metacarpal and ulnar side of base of first thumb bone.

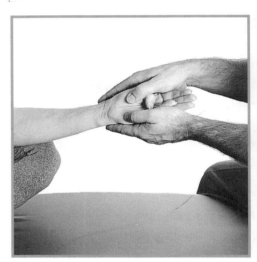

Biokinetic Exercise
Rest dorsal surface of left hand in fingers of right hand. Flex thumb toward little finger. Place right thumb over dorsal aspect of meta-carpophalangeal joint of left thumb and press towards palm.

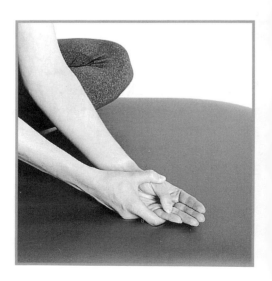

Biceps Brachii

biceps = muscle with two origins or heads; brachium = arm

Muscle Facts
Origin:
Long Head: Supraglenoidal tuberosity of scapula.
Short Head: Apex of coracoid process of the scapula.

Insertion:
Radial tuberosity and bicipital aponeurosis (into deep fascia of the forearm muscles).

Action:
Flexes and supinates forearm at the elbow.

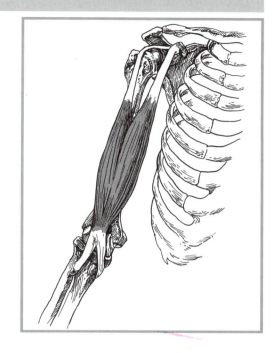

Method of Testing
Muscle Test:
Place client's elbow in the palm of your hand, flex arm 135°, palm up. For the short head start with forearm further down and slightly out.
Long Head: Pressure is at the wrist straight down.
Short Head: Pressure is at the wrist down and out.

Circuit Localize:
Long Head: Lateral half of biceps.
Short Head: Medial half of biceps.

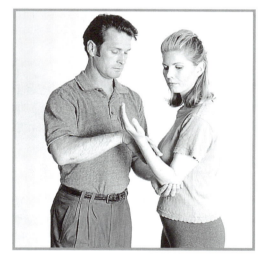

Biokinetic Exercise
Long Head:
1. Place your left palm on your left shoulder blade by reaching over your shoulder.
2. Grasp your left elbow with your right hand by reaching behind your head.
3. Push your elbow towards your left shoulder.

Short Head:
1. Fully bend your arm and hand until the back of your fingers touch your breast bone.
2. Grasp your left elbow with your right hand and push it towards your left shoulder.

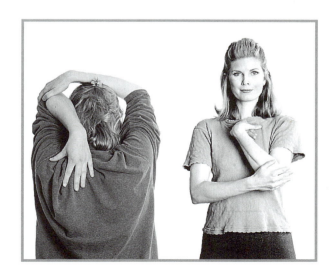

Biceps Femoris

biceps = muscle with two origins or heads; femoris = of the femur or thigh bone

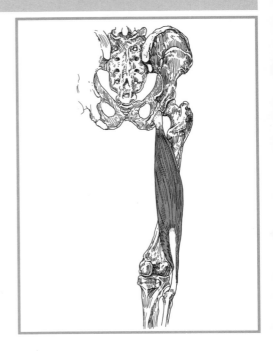

Muscle Facts
1 of the 4 muscles making up the Hamstrings
Origin:
Long Head: Medial facet of the tuberosity of the ischium and the sacrotuberous ligament.
Short Head: Lateral lip of linea aspera and lateral supracondylar line of femur.

Insertion:
Lateral side of head of fibula, lateral condyle of tibia.

Action:
Only the **long head** acts at the hip joint. It is a prime mover for extension and an assistant for lateral rotation. Both heads act as prime movers for flexion and lateral rotation at the knee.

Method of Testing
Muscle Test:
Long Head: Client prone, raise the lower leg 90° and rotate foot laterally 40°. Exert pressure in the middle of the back of the thigh to prevent cramping. Pressure is against the back of the Achilles tendon to straighten the leg.
Short Head: As above.

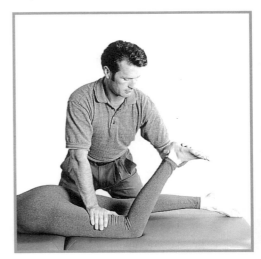

Circuit Localize:
Long Head: On the mid posterior thigh.
Short Head: On posterior lateral aspect of the thigh.

Biokinetic Exercise
For right side:
Long Head: Standing on your knees with right knee posterior 8", pull right lower leg up and out 20 degrees with right hand having weight on right knee. Push left hip towards the right.
Short Head: Standing on your knees with right knee posterior eight inches, pull lower leg up and out 20 degrees with right hand having weight on right knee.

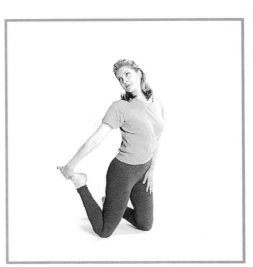

Brachioradialis

brachium = arm; radialis = of the radius

Muscle Facts

Origin:
Proximal two-thirds of lateral supracondylar ridge of humerus and lateral intermuscular septum.

Insertion:
The lateral surface of the radius at the base of the styloid process.

Action:
Flexion of the forearm at the elbow. From a position of pronation, the brachioradialis assists with supination; from a position of supination, it assists with pronation.

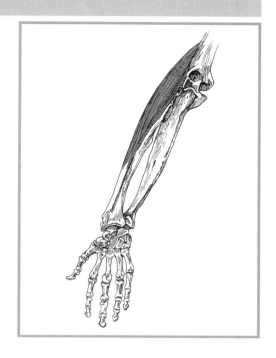

Method of Testing

Muscle Test:
The elbow is flexed with an angle of approximately 105° between the upper arm and forearm. The thumb is pointed toward the shoulder with stabilization under the elbow. Pressure is against the lower forearm in the direction of extension.

Circuit Localize:
On lateral anterior side of elbow joint.

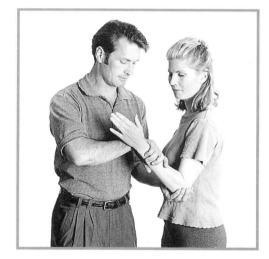

Biokinetic Exercise

1. Flex arm fully until right thumb touches right shoulder. Keep your hand straight.
2. Support elbow on lap. Then with your left hand press right hand and wrist down towards elbow and slightly towards shoulder.

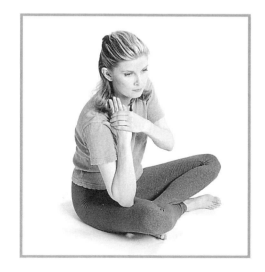

Buccinator

bucca = cheek

Muscle Facts

Origin:
Alveolar processes of maxilla and mandible and pterygomandibular raphe.

Insertion:
Orbicularis oris, angle of mouth.

Action:
Major cheek muscle; compresses cheek as in blowing air out of mouth and causes the cheeks to cave-in, producing the action of sucking.

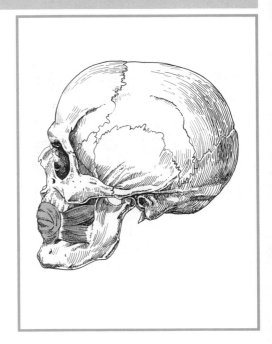

Method of Testing

Muscle Test:
Use a surrogate muscle.

Circuit Localize:
Mid to lower cheek.

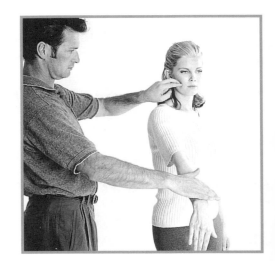

Biokinetic Exercise

Place finger inside of mouth and pull towards lower ear (top of ear for superior part of buccinator).

Coracobrachialis

*coraco = pertaining to the coracoid process on scapula;
brachium = arm*

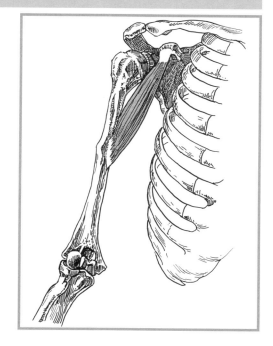

Muscle Facts
Origin:
Tip of coracoid process of scapula.

Insertion:
Antero-medial surface of the humerus, opposite the deltoid tuberosity.

Action:
Horizontal flexion and adduction of the humerus at the shoulder.

Method of Testing
Muscle Test:
With the elbow bent as far as possible, the arm 45° up and 45° from the side, stabilize the back of the shoulder. Pressure is against the end of the humerus to push the arm back and slightly out to the side.

Circuit Localize:
Four fingers below arm pit on medial side of upper arm.

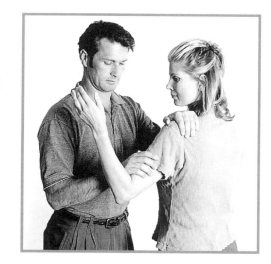

Biokinetic Exercise
1. Interlock your hands above your head keeping your arms not quite straight.
2. Turning your palms down and back, drop your head forward and permit your shoulders to sag. Rest while breathing deeply.

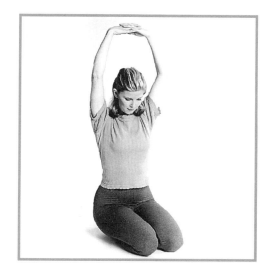

Deltoid Anterior

deltoides = triangular; anterior = front

Muscle Facts

Origin:
Anterior border and superior surface of lateral third of clavicle.

Insertion:
Deltoid tuberosity on the middle of the lateral side of the humerus.

Action:
Flexes the humerus. Assists in medial rotation and abduction.

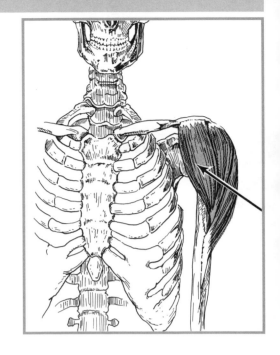

Method of Testing

Muscle Test:
With the arm straight and directly over the thigh at a 45° angle, palm down, pressure is against the distal end of the forearm to push it toward the thigh.

Circuit Localize:
On front of shoulder.

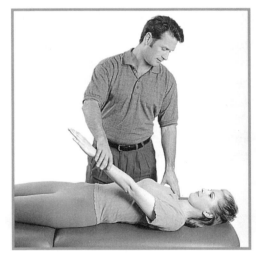

Biokinetic Exercise

1. Place your left elbow on your forehead and the back of your left hand on your chest.
2. Grasp your elbow with your right hand and compress it towards the left shoulder.
3. Arch back as far as possible. Rest.

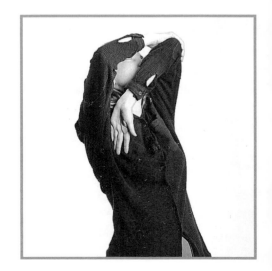

Deltoid Middle

deltoides = triangular

Muscle Facts
Origin:
Lateral margin and superior surface of acromion.

Insertion:
Deltoid tubercle on middle of the lateral side of the humerus.

Action:
A prime mover for abduction and for horizontal extension.

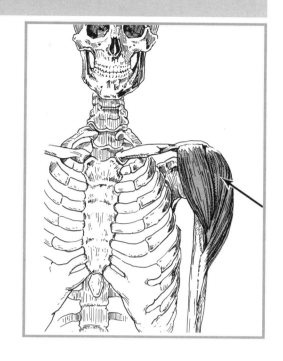

Method of Testing
Muscle Test:
With the arm abducted 90° to the side, and bent 90° at the elbow, stabilize the shoulder. Pressure is against the distal end of the humerus to bring it down to the side of the body.

Circuit Localize:
Two thumb widths below the acromion in the middleof the deltoid muscle.

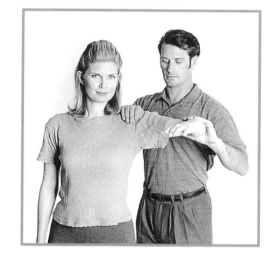

Biokinetic Exercise
1. Place your left palm on your upper back.
2. Grasp your left elbow with your right hand by reaching behind your head.
3. Push your elbow (compress) toward your left shoulder.
4. Arch back. Rest.

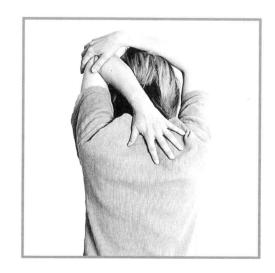

Deltoid Posterior

deltoides = triangle

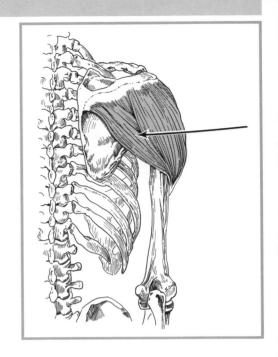

Muscle Facts

Origin:
Inferior margin of spine of scapula.

Insertion:
Deltoid tuberosity in middle of lateral side of humerus.

Action:
Abduction, horizontal extension and lateral rotation of the humerus at the shoulder.

Method of Testing

Muscle Test:
Standing or sitting, with the arm held out to the side, elbow level with the shoulder and bent 90° and the elbow drawn slightly back, pressure is downwards and forwards.

Circuit Localize:
Posterior part of deltoid muscle.

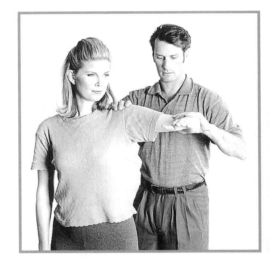

Biokinetic Exercise

1. Sit on floor.
2. Place hands pointing backwards, three feet apart and three feet behind you.
3. Lean back.
4. Rest for 30 seconds.

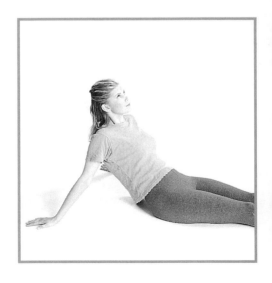

Diaphragm

dia = across; phragma = wall

Muscle Facts

Origin:
An approximately circular line passing entirely around the inner surface of the body wall. Attached to xiphoid process, costal cartilages of last six ribs interdigitating with the transversus abdominis, and anterolateral surfaces of the bodies and discs of the upper three lumbar vertebrae.

Insertion:
The central tendon, which is an oblong sheet forming the summit of the dome.

Action:
Forms floor of thoracic cavity; contraction pulls central tendon downward and increases vertical length of thorax during inspiration.

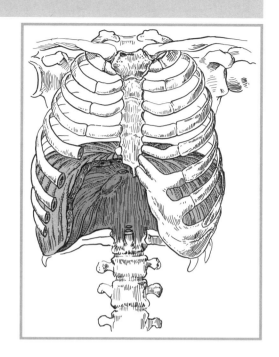

Method of Testing

Muscle Test:
Take a deep breath and hold it in. Time should be at least 40 seconds.

Or

Monitor a locked indicator muscle (IM) while breathing in and extending the abdomen to contract the diaphragm muscle. If IM unlocks diaphragm is not in balance.

Circuit Localize:
On the abdomen just left of the tip of the breast bone (xiphoid process), pushing in gently.

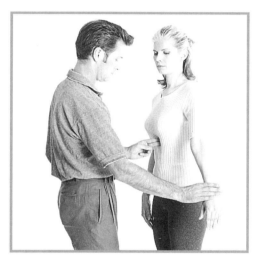

Biokinetic Exercise

1. Stand with left hand on left side of the rib cage, thumb posterior and fingers pointing anteriorly.
2. Take a deep breath, then put pressure in and up with the left hand while breathing out.
3. Bend torso anterolaterally, i.e. 45° lateral of forward.
4. Place right hand over the left hand to apply additional pressure in order to further compress the diaphragm.
5. Relax for one minute. Repeat for right side.
   OR, have a friend push on rib cage forcefully upwards and towards spine, hold for 1 minute (be careful around xiphoid, and with older people).

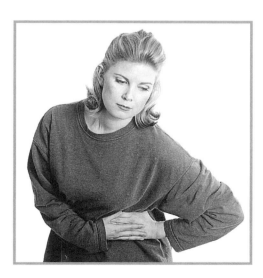

Dorsal Interossei

dorsum = back; inter = between; os = bone;

Muscle Facts
Origin:
Four dorsal interossei muscles each arise by two heads from the sides of the adjacent metatarsals.

Insertion:
Proximal end of the first phalanges and extensor expansion of the tendons of the extensor digitorum longus. The first dorsal interosseus arises from the first and second metatarsals and inserts into the medial side of the second toe. The second, third and fourth dorsal interossei insert into the lateral sides of the second, third and fourth toes.

Action:
First interosseus adducts the second toe toward the big toe. The second, third and fourth abduct the second, third and fourth toes away from the great toe. Flex the proximal and extend the middle and distal phalanges of the second, third and fourth toes.

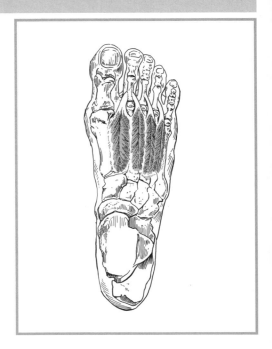

Method of Testing
Muscle Test:
Use a surrogate muscle.

Circuit Localize:
Dorsal surface of foot between metatarsals.

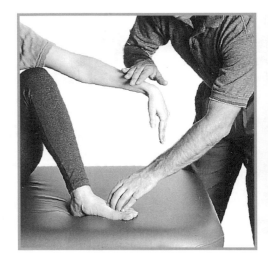

Biokinetic Exercise
1. Place fingers on underside of toes.
2. Bend toes back toward top of foot.
3. Push toes toward the metatarsal joint.

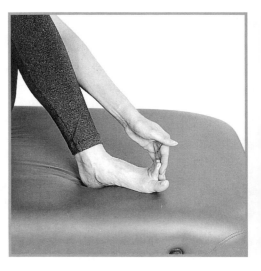

Extensor Carpi Radialis Longus

extensor = muscle which increases angle at a joint; carpus = of the wrist; radialis = of the radius; longus = long

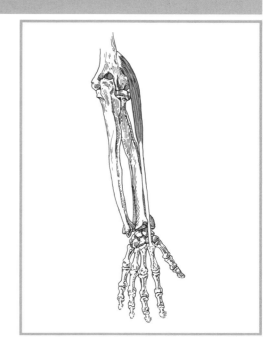

Muscle Facts
Origin:
Lateral epicondyle of humerus.

Insertion:
Dorsal surface of base of second metacarpal bone on radial side.

Action:
Extension of the wrist. Assists flexor carpi radialis in abduction (thumbward bending) at wrist.

Method of Testing
Muscle Test:
Client places forearm on table, palm down. Extend the wrist fully back on the thumb side. Pressure is on the back of the hand (thumb side) to straighten the wrist.

Circuit Localize:
Lateral side of the radius near acupuncture point Large Intestine 10, about two thumb-widths below elbow.

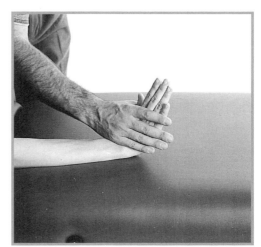

Biokinetic Exercise
1. Sitting on a chair with the elbow placed against the back of the chair, fully flex the elbow, palm up.
2. Use your other hand to extend and press the hand back towards the elbow.
3. Relax and hold position for one minute.

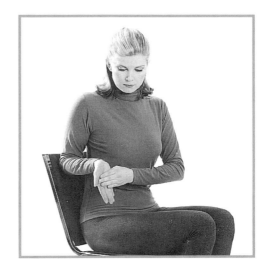

Extensor Carpi Ulnaris

extensor = muscle which increases angle at a joint; carpi = of the wrist; ulnaris = of the ulna

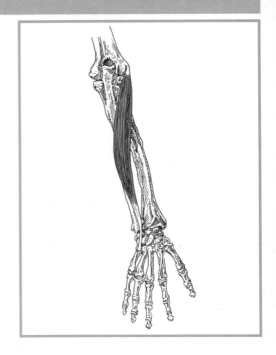

Muscle Facts

Origin:
The lateral epicondyle of the humerus and the middle third of the narrow ridge on the dorsal border of the ulna.

Insertion:
Posterior surface of base of fifth metacarpal.

Action:
Extends the wrist. Together with flexor carpi ulnaris, deviates the hand at the wrist towards the ulna.

Method of Testing

Muscle Test:
Client places palmar side of forearm on table, bending the wrist fully backwards, especially on the little finger side. Pressure is on the back of the hand (little finger side) to straighten the wrist.

Circuit Localize:
Along the posterior medial portion of the forearm.

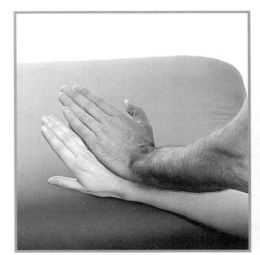

Biokinetic Exercise

1. Grasp base of the little finger and pull backwards towards the elbow.
2. Fully flex the forearm on the humerus.

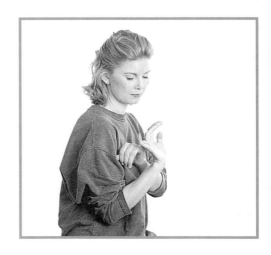

Extensor Digitorum Brevis

extensor = muscle which increases angle at a joint; digitorum = of the fingers or toes; brevis = short

Muscle Facts

Origin:
Distal dorsal and lateral surfaces of calcaneus.

Insertion:
It divides into three tendons which insert into the tendons of the extensor digitorum longus of the second, third, and fourth toes.

Action:
Extends the proximal phalanges of the second, third and fourth toes. (A fourth tendon inserts into the dorsal surface of the proximal end of the first phalanx of the great toe. This is sometimes regarded as the most medial part of extensor digitorum brevis, sometimes called extensor hallucis brevis).

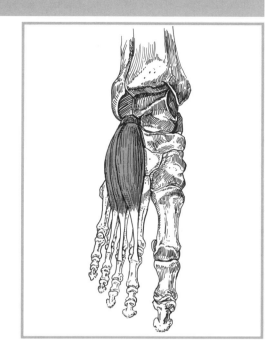

Method of Testing

Muscle Test:
Stabilize ankle in the neutral position. The person extends their toes backwards. Pressure is on the back of the proximal phalange of the second, third and fourth toes to bend them down.

Circuit Localize:
Dorsal lateral aspect of foot about two body inches anterior of base of fibula.

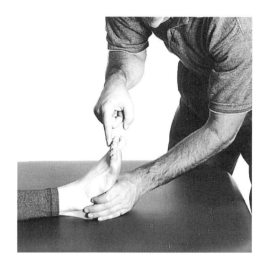

Biokinetic Exercise

1. Sit down on the edge of a chair, keeping your foot flat on the floor.
2. Bend second, third and fourth toes backwards with your hand. Rest.

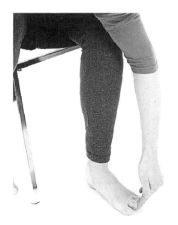

Extensor Digitorum Longus

extensor = muscle which increases angle at a joint; digitorum = of the fingers or toes; longus = long

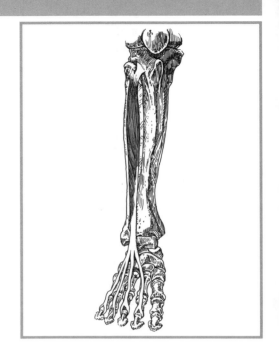

Muscle Facts

Origin:
Lateral condyle of the tibia, the upper three-fourths of the anterior surface of the fibula, and the adjacent interosseous membrane and covering deep fascia.

Insertion:
Divides into four tendons to insert into the dorsal aspects of the middle and distal phalanges of the four outer toes.

Action:
Extends the outer four toes. Dorsiflexes and everts foot at the ankle.

Method of Testing

Muscle Test:
Stabilize ankle in the neutral position. The client dorsiflexes their toes as much as possible. Pressure is on the back of the middle and distal phalanges of the second, third and fourth toes to bend them down.

Circuit Localize:
Two-thirds of the way up the front of the lower leg immediately lateral to the tibialis anterior muscle, over the fibula.

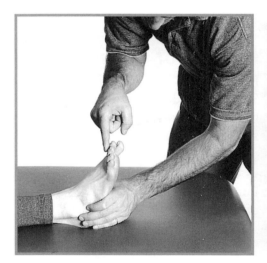

Biokinetic Exercise

1. Sit down on the edge of a chair, keeping your foot flat on the floor.
2. Bring the foot back under the chair as far as possible while still keeping the heel on the floor.
3. Bend your toes backwards with your hand. Rest.

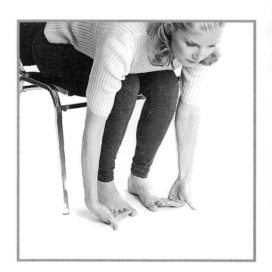

Extensor Hallucis Brevis

extensor = muscle which increases angle at a joint; hallucis = of the great toe; brevis = short

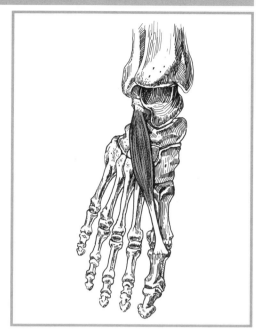

Muscle Facts
the medial section of the extensor digitorum brevis

Origin:
The distal lateral dorsal aspect of the calcaneus, and the adjacent ligaments.

Insertion:
The dorsal surface of the base of the proximal phalanx of the great toe.

Action:
Extends proximal phalanx of the great toe.

Method of Testing
Muscle Test:
Have ankle in the neutral position. Stabilize the ankle so that tibialis anterior isn't recruited. Bend great toe back towards shin bone. Pressure is on the proximal phalanx of the great toe to bend it down and in towards the other foot.

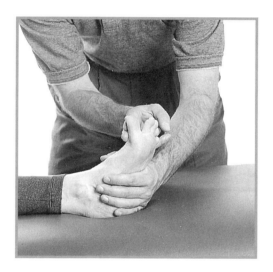

Circuit Localize:
Into middle of dorsal aspect of foot half way between outer ankle bone and proximal end of great toe.

Biokinetic Exercise
In seated position hold feet in neutral position. Bring arms down on outside of knees, grasp great toes, and pull back towards outer ankle bones.

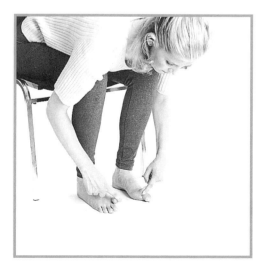

Extensor Hallucis Longus

extensor = muscle which increases angle at a joint; hallucis = of the great toe; longus = long

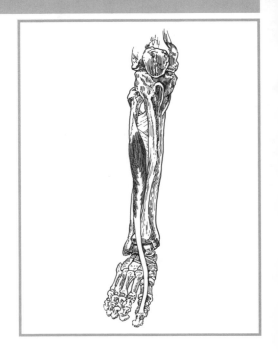

Muscle Facts

Origin:
Middle half of the anterior surface of the fibula and the adjacent interosseous membrane.

Insertion:
Dorsal surface of base of distal phalanx of the great toe.

Action:
Extends the distal phalanx of the great toe. Continued action extends proximal phalanx and dorsiflexes and inverts the foot at the ankle.

Method of Testing

Muscle Test:
Have ankle in the neutral position. Stabilize the ankle to prevent tibialis anterior involvement. Bend great toe up. Pressure is on top of the great toe to bend it forward.

Circuit Localize:
Middle of anterior lower leg between tibia and fibula.

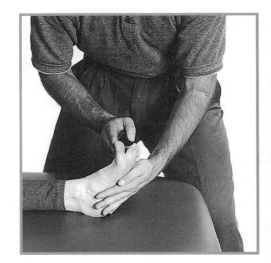

Biokinetic Exercise

1. Sit down on the edge of a chair, keeping your foot flat on the floor.
2. Bring the foot back under the chair as far as possible while keeping the heel on the floor.
3. Bend your great toe backwards as far as you can. Rest.

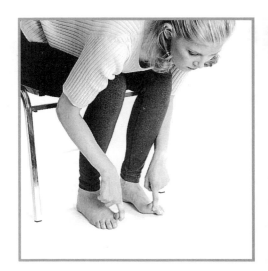

Extensor Pollicis Longus

extensor = muscle which increases angle at a joint; pollicis = of the thumb; longus = long

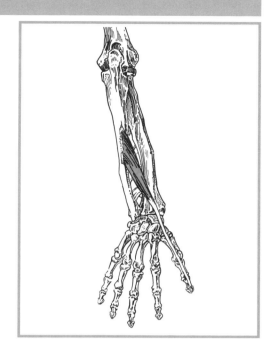

Muscle Facts
Origin:
Posterior surface of the middle third of the ulna and the interosseus membrane.

Insertion:
The dorsal surface of the base of the distal phalanx of the thumb.

Action:
Extends the distal phalanx of the thumb. Continued action, extends proximal phalanx and metacarpal, and adducts the first metacarpal, drawing the thumb into the plane of the rest of the hand.

Method of Testing
Muscle Test:
With the forearm on a table, fully extend the thumb. Pressure is on the thumb to flex it.

Circuit Localize:
One-third of way up the dorsal surface of the forearm between ulna and radius.

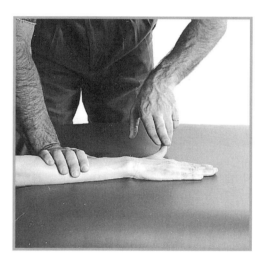

Biokinetic Exercise
Grasp palmar surface of thumb and pull backwards towards elbow.

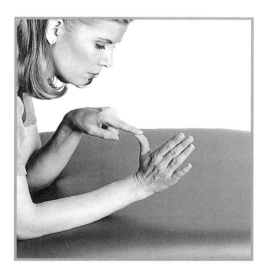

External Oblique

external = outer, closer to the surface; oblique = muscle fibers running diagonally to midline of body

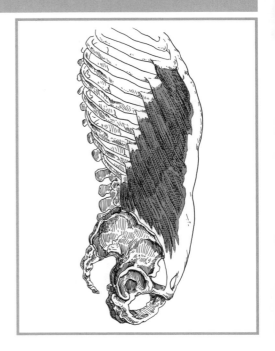

Muscle Facts
Origin:
External surfaces and inferior borders of the 5-12th ribs by tendinous slips that interdigitate with the serratus anterior and latissimus dorsi.

Insertion:
Anterior half of outer lip of iliac crest. Inguinal ligament. Linea alba ("white line") by means of the broad abdominal aponeurosis from xiphoid process to crest of pubis.

Action:
Acting unilaterally, rotates trunk to the opposite side, and flexes it laterally on the side of muscle contraction. Acting bilaterally, flexes the trunk anteriorly, supports and compresses the abdominal organs, giving anterior support to the spinal column. Gives anterior stabilization to pelvis.

Method of Testing
Muscle Test:
Client sits with knees bent and together, hands on the opposite shoulders, and leaning back, chin-up. To test left side, left shoulder is rotated forwards. Practitioner holds client's shoulders and attempts to rotate to the left and back simultaneously. **Or,** client lies on back, both legs raised 80°. Stabilize left shoulder, and press ankles down and to right away from left shoulder.

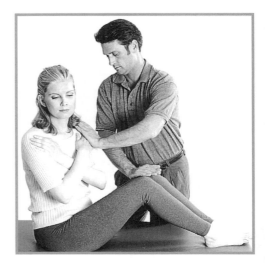

Circuit Localize:
Four thumb widths lateral of navel, grasping superficial muscles between fingers and thumb.

Biokinetic Exercise
For Left Side:
1. Sit on the floor with your legs bent under and to the sides.
2. With your left arm crossing your front, grasp your right heel and bend your left shoulder down and to the right until it touches or almost touches your right knee.
3. Twist to the right. Rest.

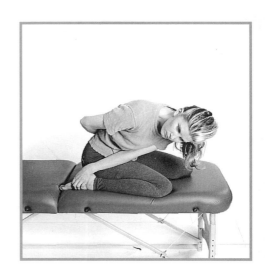

Flexor Carpi Radialis

flexor = muscle which decreases angle at a joint; carpi = of the wrist; radialis = of the radius

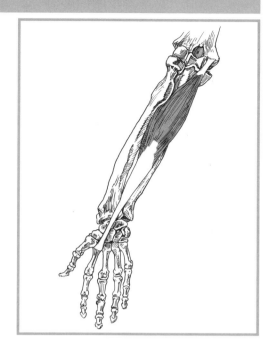

Muscle Facts
Origin:
Medial epicondyle of humerus.

Insertion:
Anterior surface of base of second (and sometimes third) metacarpal(s).

Action:
Flexes and abducts the wrist.

Method of Testing
Muscle Test:
Client places forearm on table, fully flexing wrist so fingers point towards inner elbow. Apply pressure to radial side of client's palm in an attempt to extend the hand.

Circuit Localize:
Two thumbs below elbow on anterior midline for forearm.

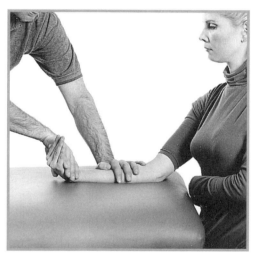

Biokinetic Exercise
1. Sit in a chair, place the back of the fingers of your left hand into your left armpit.
2. Support your elbow on your thigh.
3. Press the back of your hand near the index finger towards your elbow with your right hand.

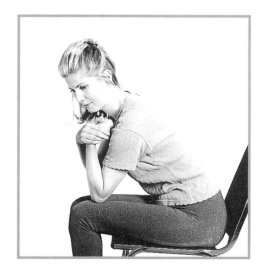

Flexor Carpi Ulnaris

flexor = muscle which decreases angle at a joint; carpi = of the wrist; ulnaris = of the ulna

Muscle Facts

Origin:
Medial epicondyle of humerus, medial margin of the olecranon and upper two-thirds of the dorsal border of the ulna.

Insertion:
The palmar surfaces of the pisiform and hamate bones and of the fifth metacarpal.

Action:
Flexes the wrist joint. Adducts the wrist medially (ulnar deviation) together with extensor carpi ulnaris.

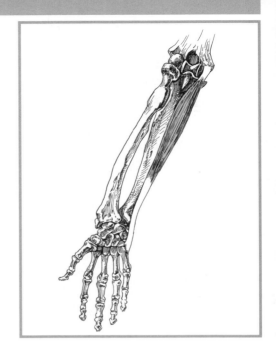

Method of Testing

Muscle Test:
Client places forearm on table palm up. Flex palm towards elbow as much as possible. Stabilize arm. Pressure is against 5th metacarpal area of palm to extend it.

Circuit Localize:
Two thumbs below elbow on the medial side of forearm.

Biokinetic Exercise

1. Bring your left palm near your face, elbow down.
2. Twist your palm outward so that little finger is near the shoulder.
3. Place the palm of the right hand on the back of the left hand and continue to twist left hand (palm) outward.
4. Palmar flex wrist of left hand about 45°.

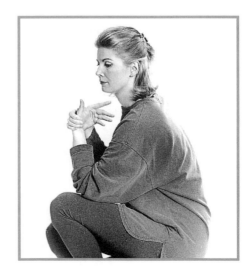

Flexor Digitorum Brevis

flexor = muscle which decreases angle at a joint; digitorum = of the fingers or toes; brevis = short

Muscle Facts

Origin:
Medial process of tuberosity of the calcaneus, central part of the plantar aponeurosis.

Insertion:
By four tendons that divide into two slips that insert into the sides of the middle phalanges of the second through fifth toes.

Action:
Plantar flexes the middle phalanges on the proximal phalanges, continued action flexes the proximal phalanges on the metatarsals.

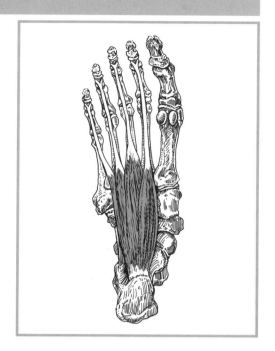

Method of Testing

Muscle Test:
The client bends the toes down at the first joint. Pressure is under the toes to straighten them.

Circuit Localize:
In line between the middle of the heel and the second to fifth toes in the middle of the plantar surface of foot.

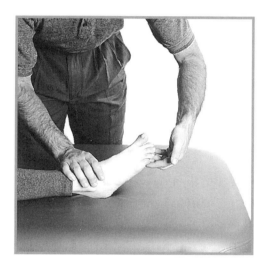

Biokinetic Exercise

1. Sit in a chair, place your left foot on your right thigh.
2. Grasp the top of your foot near the base of the toes and press it towards the bottom of the heel.
3. Press the heel towards the bottom of the toes.

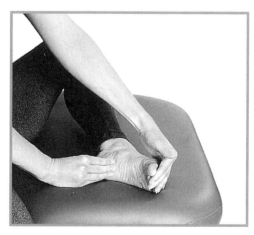

Flexor Digitorum Longus

flexor = muscle which decreases angle at a joint; digitorum = of the fingers or toes; longus = long

Muscle Facts

Origin:
Posterior surface of much of middle and upper tibia.

Insertion:
Divides into four tendons that insert on the plantar surfaces of bases of distal phalanges of the second through fifth toes. Each tendon passes through an opening in the corresponding tendon of the flexor digitorum brevis.

Action:
Prime mover for flexion of the second through fifth toes. Assists with plantar flexion and inversion of the foot at the ankle.

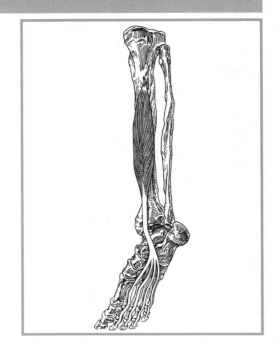

Method of Testing

Muscle Test:
Client bends tips of toes down. Pressure is from under the toes to straighten them.

Circuit Localize:
Along medial side of lower leg behind tibia.

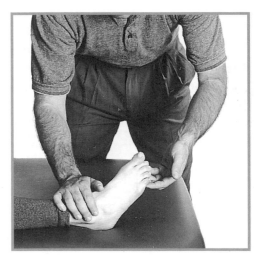

Biokinetic Exercise

1. Sit on the edge of a chair and fold your feet under so that you are stepping on the tops of your feet near the second through fifth toes.
2. Put your knees about two feet apart and your heels back.
3. Gently press down on your feet.

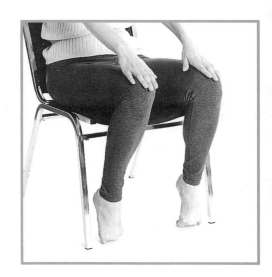

Flexor Digitorum Profundus

flexor = muscle which decreases angle at a joint; digitorum = of the fingers or toes; profundus = deep

Muscle Facts

Origin:
The upper three-fourths of the anterior and medial surfaces of the ulna, ulnar half of interosseous membrane, aponeurosis from upper three-fourths of dorsal border of ulna, medial side of coronoid process.

Insertion:
By four tendons which separate after passing the wrist and go to the four fingers. Each tendon passes through the split in the corresponding flexor digitorum superficialis tendon and is inserted into the palmar surface of the base of the distal phalanx.

Action:
Flexes fingers primarily at distal interphalangeal joint. Assists in flexing at wrist and other joints of fingers.

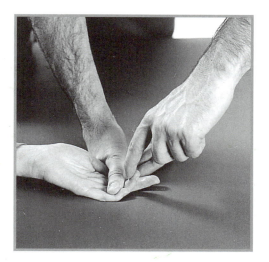

Method of Testing

Muscle Test:
Wrist in neutral position with palm up, fingertip only bent. Stabilize the first two bones of the finger. Pressure is on the finger tip to straighten it.

Circuit Localize:
Deep about two inches distal from elbow joint on medial half of anterior forearm.

Biokinetic Exercise

1. Sit down and place the back of your knuckles on the outer side of your biceps, palm down.
2. Press the top of your hand down towards your elbow.

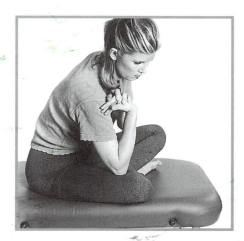

Flexor Digitorum Superficialis – sublimis

flexor = muscle which decreases angle at a joint; digitorum = of the fingers or toes; superficialis = superficial

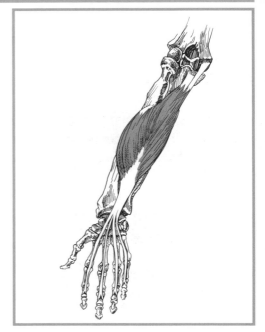

Muscle Facts

Origin:
Deep Head (Radial Head): Oblique line of the radius extending from the radial tuberosity to the insertion of the pronator teres.
Superficial Head (Humero-Ulnar Head): Medial epicondyle of the humerus by the common flexor tendon, ulnar collateral ligament of the elbow and the coronoid process of ulna.

Insertion:
Deep Head: To index and little finger.
Superficial Head: To middle two fingers. Four tendons separate after passing the wrist and go to the four fingers. Opposite the proximal phalanx each tendon splits into two parts, which are inserted into the sides of the base of the middle phalanx. The flexor digitorum profundus tendon passes between the two slips of flexor digitorum superficialis on its way to the finger tip.

Action:
Flexes the middle phalanx of each finger on the proximal phalanx. Continued action, flexes the proximal phalanx at the hand, flexes the hand at the wrist.

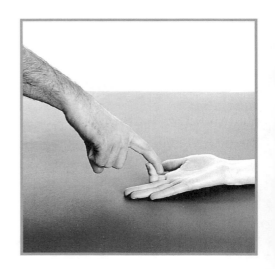

Method of Testing

Muscle Test:
With arm on table, palm up, bend finger at the first joint. Pressure is against middle phalanx of the finger to attempt to straighten it.

Circuit Localize:
Middle of anterior aspect of forearm.

Biokinetic Exercise

1. Sit down and place the dorsal surface of the fingers of your right hand on the biceps of your right arm.
2. Flexing your wrist fully, press the top of your hand towards your elbow as it rests upon your right thigh.

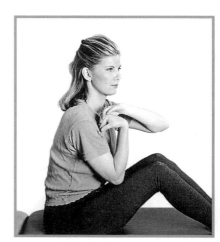

Flexor Hallucis Brevis

flexor = muscle which decreases angle at a joint; hallucis = of the great toe; brevis = short

Muscle Facts

Origin:
Medial part of the plantar surface of the cuboid bone, adjacent part of the lateral cuneiform bone.

Insertion:
The tendon divides, being inserted on medial and lateral sides of the base of the proximal phalanx of the great toe.

Action:
Flexes the proximal phalanx of the great toe.

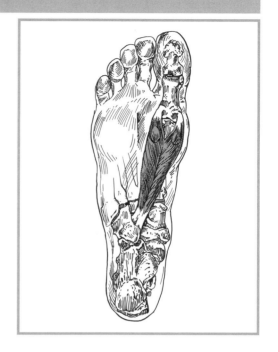

Method of Testing

Muscle Test:
Support the foot in a neutral position, leaving the joint at the junction of the foot and great toe free to move. The client bends the toe down at this joint while keeping the toe straight. Press against the under surface of the great toe to straighten it.

Circuit Localize:
On plantar surface of foot along first metatarsal.

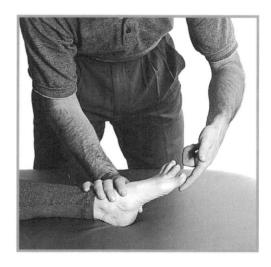

Biokinetic Exercise

Plantar flex the foot. Press the top base of the great toe towards the bottom of the heel.

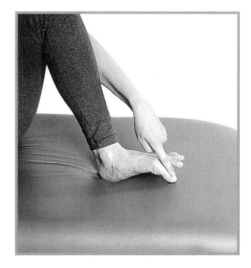

Flexor Hallucis Longus

flexor = muscle which decreases angle at a joint; hallucis = of the great toe; longus = long

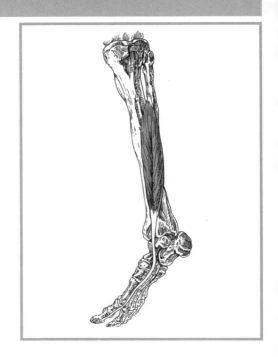

Muscle Facts
Origin:
Distal two-thirds of posterior surface of fibula and the lowest part of the interosseous membrane.

Insertion:
Plantar surface of base of distal phalanx of the great toe.

Action:
Flexes great toe toward sole of foot. Aids in plantar flexion and inversion of the foot at the ankle. Helps stabilize the medial ankle.

Method of Testing
Muscle Test:
Foot in neutral position. Support the joint between the great toe and the foot. The testee holds the tip of the great toe bent down. Pressure is against the under surface of the toe to straighten it.

Circuit Localize:
Just lateral of the mid-posterior line of the lower leg in the lower one-third of the leg.

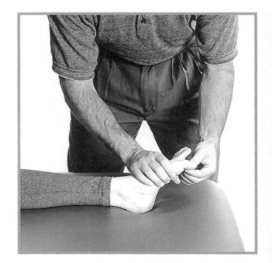

Biokinetic Exercise
1. Sit in a chair. Pass the left arm outside of the left thigh, under the knee and inside of the lower leg. Raise knee to chest.
2. Plantar flex the foot, grasp the top of the great toe at its base and pull towards the heel and towards the outside of the left hip. Keep the foot in a line with the lower leg.

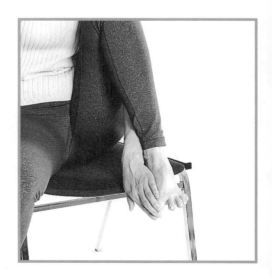

Flexor Pollicis Brevis

flexor = muscle which decreases angle at a joint; pollicis = of the thumb; brevis = short

Muscle Facts
Origin:
Superficial Head: Distal border of flexor retinaculum and crest of trapezium bone.
Deep Head: Trapezoid and capitate bones of the wrist, palmar ligaments of the distal row of carpal bones.

Insertion:
The outer more superficial portion of the muscle inserts into radial side of the base of the proximal phalanx of the thumb. The very small inner deeper portion of the muscle inserts into ulnar side of base of proximal phalanx of thumb with adductor pollicis.

Action:
Abduction and medial rotation of the proximal phalanx and the metacarpal of the thumb.

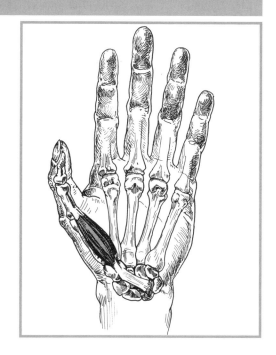

Method of Testing
Muscle Test:
Stabilize hand. Flex thumb at its first joint to bring it across towards little finger. Pressure is on proximal phalanx of thumb to extend it.

Circuit Localize:
Medial surface of fleshy pad of thumb.

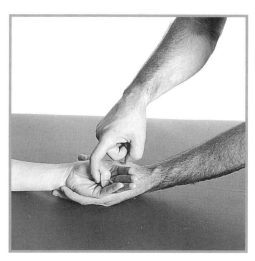

Biokinetic Exercise
1. Bring tip of thumb across to base of little finger.
2. Use other hand to press thumb towards little finger side of the hand.

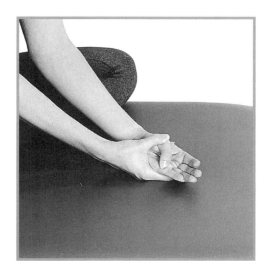

Flexor Pollicis Longus

flexor = muscle which decreases angle at a joint; pollicis = of the thumb; longus = long

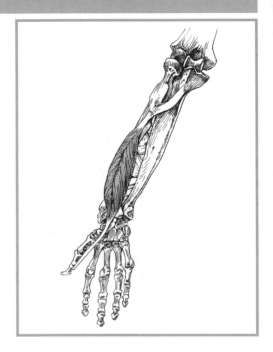

Muscle Facts

Origin:
Anterior surface of middle half of radius. Adjacent interosseous membrane and a slip from the coronoid process of the ulna or medial epicondyle of humerus.

Insertion:
Plantar surface of base of distal phalanx of the thumb.

Action:
Flexes the distal phalanx of the thumb. Continued action flexes the proximal phalanx and flexes and adducts the metacarpal and wrist.

Method of Testing

Muscle Test:
Stabilize the thumb with the last joint bent. Press against the thumb tip to attempt to straighten it.

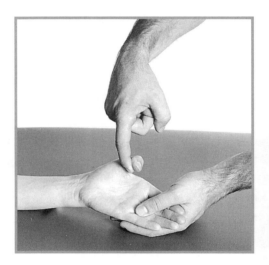

Circuit Localize:
Mid-forearm, lateral side of anterior surface. Three thumbs distal of elbow joint deep in lateral side of ulna (ulnar head). On medial side of radius (humeral head).

Biokinetic Exercise

Flex wrist fully. Push side of thumb in toward wrist.

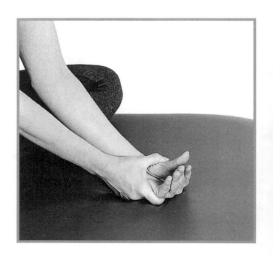

54

Gastrocnemius

gaster = belly; kneme = leg

Muscle Facts
Origin:
Lateral Head: Lateral condyle and posterior surface of femur.
Medial Head: Medial condyle and adjacent part of femur.

Insertion:
Posterior surface of calcaneus by way of the achilles tendon.

Action:
A prime mover for plantar flexion. Assists with knee flexion. Stabilizes the femur on the tibia.

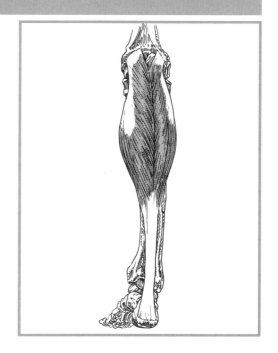

Method of Testing
Muscle Test:
Start with the knee flexed 40° (angle between posterior thigh and lower leg of 140°) and the foot in plantar flexion. Pressure is against the distal part of the dorsal surface of the lower leg to straighten the leg while the knee is stabilized.
Or
Client lies facedown with knees straight and leg slightly raised. Toes are pointed and pressure is at the ball of the foot tostraighten to a normal position.

Circuit Localize:
Into posterior belly of lower leg.

Biokinetic Exercise
Sitting on floor with legs folded back to sides, grasp your heels and forcibly press them forward towards inside of knees. Lean back.

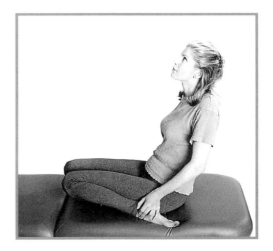

Gluteus Maximus

gloutos = buttock; maximus = largest

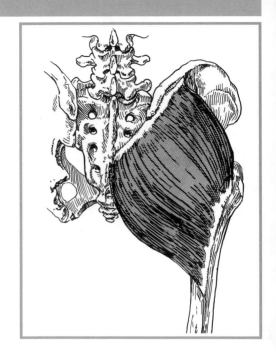

Muscle Facts

Origin:
Posterior gluteal line of ilium; posterior surface of lower part of sacrum and side of coccyx; posterior surface of sacrotuberous ligament and aponeurosis of erector spinae.

Insertion:
A rough line about four inches long on the posterior aspect of the femur between the greater trochanter and the linea aspera, and the iliotibial tract of the fascia lata.

Action:
Extends thigh at the hip. Assists in laterally rotating the thigh. The upper two-thirds of the muscle assists with abduction, especially when the weight of the body falls onto one limb, as in running.

Method of Testing

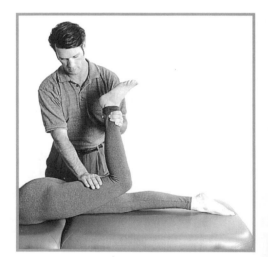

Muscle Test:
Lying face down with the knee flexed 90° and leg raised up. Pressure is against the thigh to push it back down, keeping the knee bent.

Circuit Localize:
Mid fleshy part of buttocks.

Biokinetic Exercise

1. Kneel on your knees, turning your right leg out 60°, keeping your knees together.
2. Reach back with your left hand and grasp your right heel, arching back and twist to the left. Rest while breathing deeply. MOVE SLOWLY. (You may need to ask someone to hold you in this position).

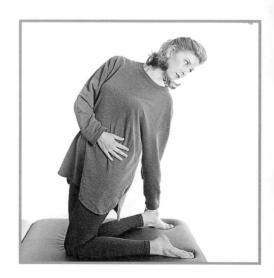

Gluteus Medius

gloutos = buttock; medius = middle

Muscle Facts

Origin: The outer surface of the ilium near its crest between the posterior gluteal line above and the anterior gluteal line below; also the gluteal aponeurosis.

Insertion: Oblique ridge on lateral surface of greater trochanter.

Action: Abducts and medially rotates thigh. Muscle's major function seems to be relatively static contraction in order to prevent hip adduction when the opposite leg is lifted during locomotion.

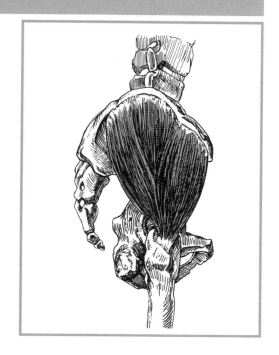

Method of Testing

Muscle Test: Client lies on back. Bring the leg straight out to the side with the pelvis stabilized. Pressure is against the ankle to bring it towards the midline.

Circuit Localize: Midway between lateral surface of ilium and greater trochanter of femur.

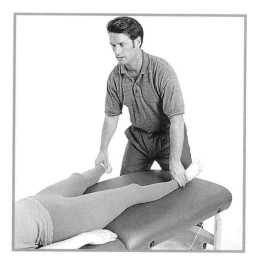

Biokinetic Exercise

For left side:
1. Standing with feet two feet apart, turn the left foot in 100°.
2. Press left thigh forward and to the right with the left hand. Rest.

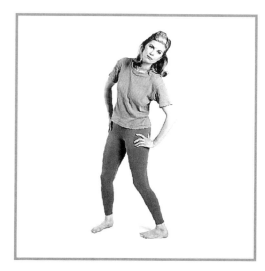

Gluteus Minimus

gloutos = buttock; minimus = smallest

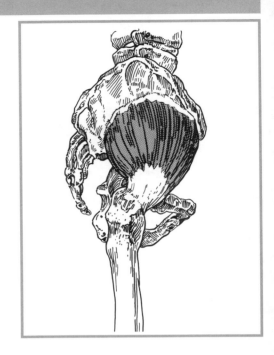

Muscle Facts

Origin:
Outer surface of ilium between anterior and inferior gluteal lines, and margin of greater sciatic notch.

Insertion:
Anterior aspect of greater trochanter of femur.

Action:
Abducts femur at the hip and rotates it medially. Assists in hip flexion.

Method of Testing

Muscle Test:
Client on side, raise leg 30° and rotate foot until it points down 45°. Stabilize torso and press lower leg down and slightly posterior.

Circuit Localize:
Deeply on upper mid lateral side of buttocks.

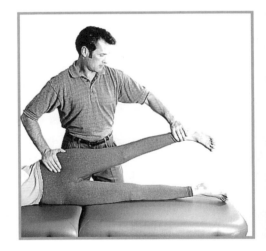

Biokinetic Exercise

Dead frog position: Lay on your back, put your knees far out to the sides and the soles of your feet together. Place your heels about one foot from your groin.

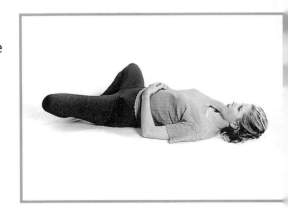

Gracilis

gracilis = slender

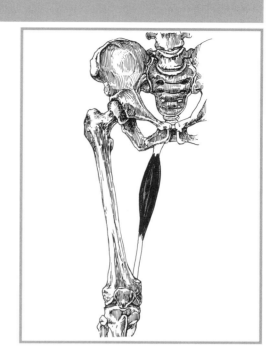

Muscle Facts
Origin:
Anterior margins of the lower half of the symphysis pubis and upper half of the pubic arch.

Insertion:
Medial surface of the tibia below the condyle.

Action:
Adduction at the hip joint. Assists with flexion and medial rotation of the thigh. At the knee, assists with flexion and medial rotation of the tibia.
Reversed Origin-Insertion Action: When the thigh is fixed, flexes pelvis at the hip.

Method of Testing
Muscle Test:
Lying face down with the knee bent about 45°. Stabilizing the knee with one hand, pressure is against the inside of the ankle to push the foot out to the side. **Or**, lying face up client raises their straight leg slightly and medially rotates it, so their foot is on top of the other foot. Pressure is against the ankle to pull it out in abduction, while stabilizing the other leg.

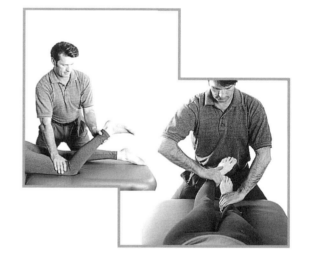

Circuit Localize:
The medial side of the thigh.

Biokinetic Exercise
1. Kneel upright and place your left knee eight inches behind your right knee. Keep your legs together.
2. Bring your left heel up to your right buttocks with your right hand.
3. Arch back with your hips forward and put your weight on your left knee.
4. Rest while breathing deeply.

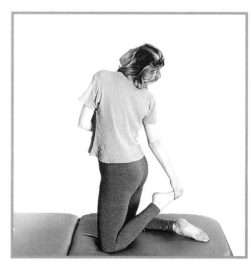

Iliacus

iliacus = pertaining to the ilium

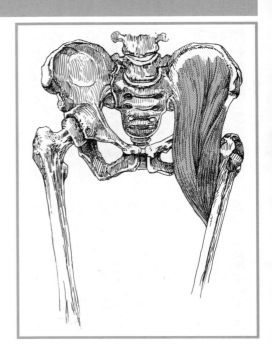

Muscle Facts
Origin:
Superior two-thirds of the iliac fossa; inner lip of iliac crest; base of the sacrum.

Insertion:
Lateral side of tendon of psoas major muscle. Shaft of femur about an inch below and in front of the lesser trochanter.

Action:
Hip joint flexion and stabilization.
Reversed Origin-Insertion Action: When the thigh is fixed, the iliacus muscle flexes the pelvis on the thigh, as in rising to a sitting position from the supine position.

Method of Testing
Muscle Test:
Lying face down: Flex the knee to 90° and rotate the femur medially as far as possible. Pressure is at the ankle to bring it toward the midline, while stabilizing the knee.

Circuit Localize:
Press in very deeply medially and just inferior to the origin of the sartorius muscle, inferior to the anterior superior crest of the ilium.

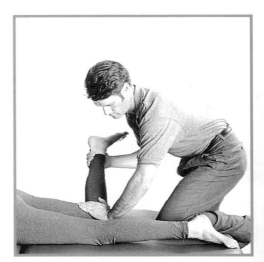

Biokinetic Exercise
1. Sit on the floor in a tailor fashion, ankles crossing each other.
2. Bend forwards and rest for one minute.
3. Bend toward your left knee and rest for one minute. While in the resting position, pull the left knee toward your hips.

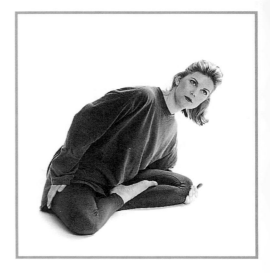

Infraspinatus

infra = below; spinatus = spine of scapula

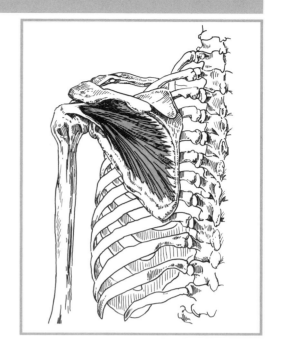

Muscle Facts

Origin:
Medial two-thirds of the fossa inferior to spine of scapula.

Insertion:
On posterior aspect of middle of greater tubercle of humerus.

Action:
Rotates humerus laterally and helps to retain humerus in shoulder joint.

Method of Testing

Muscle Test:
Extend arm out to side, palm down. Bend the elbow to a 90° angle. Rotate forearm down about 20°. Place one hand under elbow to stabilize it and the other hand on the wrist to rotate it down and back.

Circuit Localize:
In line midway between infraspinous fossa of scapula and the greater tubercle of humerus.

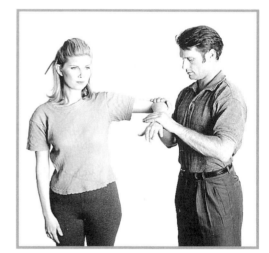

Biokinetic Exercise

1. Kneel. Clasp your hands together behind you, and turn them back and down.
2. Bow your head down to your knees and bring your rear end up.
3. Raise your clasped hands up over your head and forward, keeping your arms straight.

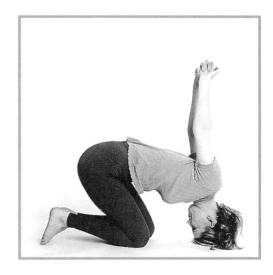

Internal Oblique

internal = inner; oblique = muscle fibers running diagonally to midline of body

Muscle Facts

Origin:
Lateral half of inguinal ligament, anterior two-thirds of middle lip of iliac crest, and posterior layer of the thoracolumbar fascia.

Insertion:
Crest of the pubis and the linea alba by its aponeurosis. Cartilages of last three or four ribs.

Action:
Acting unilaterally, rotates the trunk toward the side of contraction, and laterally flexes the trunk on that same side. Acting bilaterally, flexes the vertebral column bringing the anterior thorax and pelvis closer together. Supports and compresses the abdominal organs.

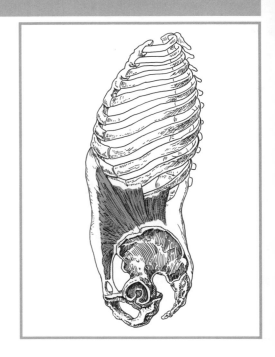

Method of Testing

Muscle Test:
For left side: Client sits with knees bent and together, hands on the opposite shoulders, leaning back slightly, chin up. Left shoulder is rotated forwards. Stabilize the upper legs. Pressure is against the left shoulder to push it through the line of the shoulders.

Circuit Localize:
Grasp deeply on lateral side muscles of abdomen.

Biokinetic Exercise

1. Sitting on the floor, bring your right arm across your front and hold on to your left buttocks.
2. With the right hand pull yourself around to the left.
3. Now lean forward and to the left side bringing the right shoulder close to the ground. Rest while breathing deeply.

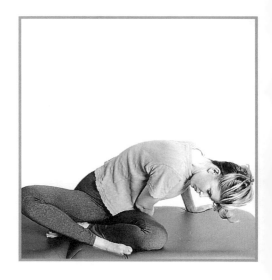

Latissimus Dorsi

latissimus = widest; dorsi = of the back

Muscle Facts
Origin:
Spines of lower six thoracic vertebrae, lumbar vertebrae, crests of sacrum and ilium, lower four ribs; usually a few fibers from inferior angle of scapula.

Insertion:
Inferior aspect of intertubercular groove of humerus.

Action:
Extends, adducts, and rotates arm medially; draws shoulder downward and backward.

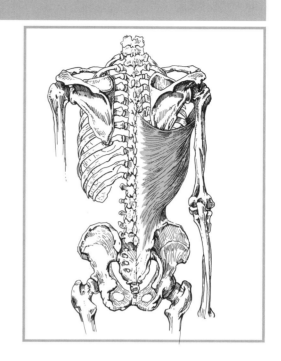

Method of Testing
Muscle Test:
Client places arm close in to side of body rotated medially so that the palm faces outwards. Be sure elbow is straight. Practitioner attempts to press arm straight out to the side, away from body.

Circuit Localize:
Grasp, between thumb and finger tips, that portion of the **muscle** in the lower back inferior to the rib cage. For the **tendon** point into the lower back about an inch lateral to the lumbar vertebrae (in Biokinesiology the tendon has been related to blood sugar imbalances).

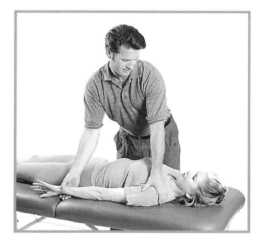

Biokinetic Exercise
1. Kneel upright, bring your right foot up behind you and grasp it with your left hand on the outside of the right foot.
2. Arch back, turning far to the left, pull your shoulder down and back towards your right foot. Rest for 30 seconds (one minute for the tendon). If this position is too difficult, it can be done lying face down.

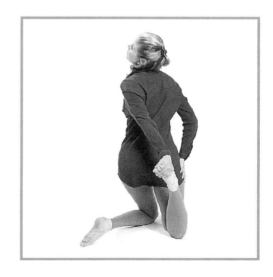

Levator Scapulae

levator = lifter; scapulae = of the shoulder blade

Muscle Facts

Origin:
Transverse processes of first four cervical vertebrae.

Insertion:
Vertebral (medial) border of scapula between superior angle and scapular spine.

Action:
Prime mover for elevation of the shoulder girdle. In erect standing, with the arm dangling downward, contraction of levator scapula allows the scapula to rotate so the glenoid cavity faces inferiorly.

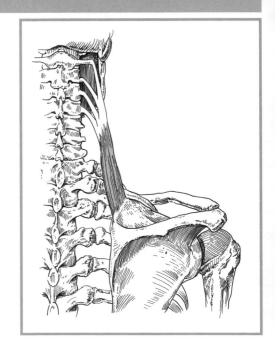

Method of Testing

Muscle Test:
Have client bend sideways so that bent elbow is against side of hip. Hold the shoulder down as you attempt to pull the elbow away from the side. Have the person keep their opposite arm away from their side to avoid recruiting the opposite rhomboid.

Circuit Localize:
In line, fairly deep, midway between the second cervical and the scapula.

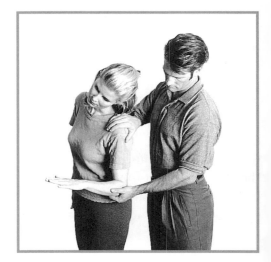

Biokinetic Exercise

For Left Side:
1. Sit on the floor with your legs comfortably in front of you, placing your hands together behind you with your fingers pointing back.
2. Lean and arch back, facing up to the ceiling.
3. Tilt your head 45° to the left.

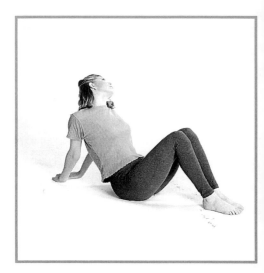

Lumbricals – of the foot

lumbricus = earthworm

Muscle Facts

Origin:
From two adjacent tendons of the flexor digitorum longus, except the first which arises from the medial side of the first tendon of the flexor digitorum longus.

Insertion:
On the medial side of the proximal phalanx of the 2nd-5th toes, into the dorsal expansions of the tendons to the extensor digitorum longus.

Action:
Flexes the 2-5th toes downward at the metatarsalphalangeal joints, extends the interphalangeal joints.

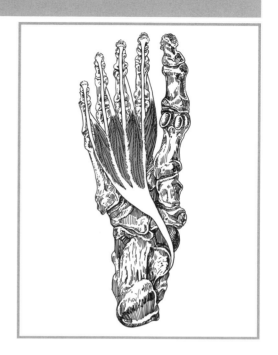

Method of Testing

Muscle Test:
The foot is stabilized close to the toes. The toes are held down. Pressure is under the first phalanges of the toes to straighten them (keep the other joints straight).

Circuit Localize:
Bottom of the foot between the metatarsals.

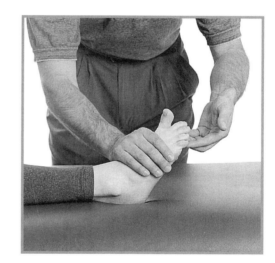

Biokinetic Exercise

1. With the right thumb, compress the middle of the sole of the left foot toward the second toe.
2. At the same time, with the left hand press the first phalanx of the second toe toward the middle of the foot. Rest.
3. Repeat for third, fourth and fifth toes.

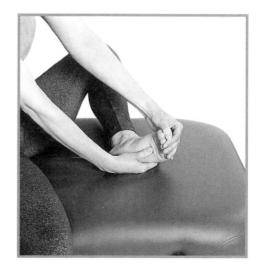

Lumbricals – of the hand

lumbricus = earthworm

Muscle Facts

Origin:
Tendons of flexor digitorum profundus in center of palm.

Insertion:
On the radial side of the base of the proximal row of phalanges into the extensor expansion.

Action:
Principal extensors of the interphalangeal joints in association with the extensor digitorum. Weak flexors of the metacarpophalangeal joints.

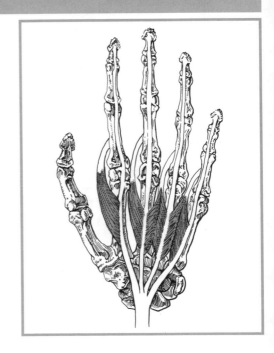

Method of Testing

Muscle Test:
Client places forearm on table. The fingers are straight but flexed at the metacarpophalangeal joint. Stabilize lower forearm with one hand. Pressure is under the base of the fingers to extend them one by one.

Circuit Localize:
Between the metacarpal bones.

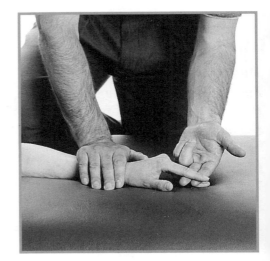

Biokinetic Exercise

1. Bring the back of your hand up to your biceps, resting your elbow on your thigh with palm down.
2. Individually press the thumb side of each finger toward the heel of your hand.

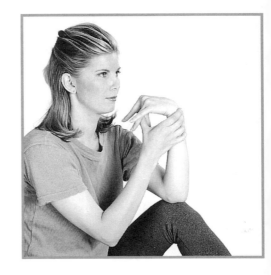

Masseter

maseter = one that chews

Muscle Facts
Origin:
Superficial portion: Zygomatic process of maxilla. Anterior two-thirds of inferior border of zygomatic arch.
Deep portion: Posterior third of inferior border of zygomatic arch. Whole medial surface of zygomatic arch.

Insertion:
Superficial portion: Angle and lower half of lateral surface of ramus of mandible.
Deep portion: Lateral surface of superior half of ramus of mandible. Lateral surface of coronoid process.

Action:
Elevates mandible as in closing the mouth and protracts (protrudes) mandible.

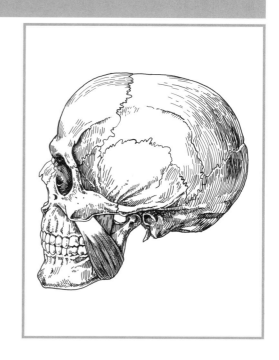

Method of Testing
Muscle Test:
Use a surrogate muscle.

Circuit Localize:
In line, between zygomatic arch and ramus of jaw.

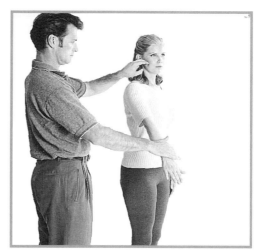

Biokinetic Exercise
Massage down from the zygomatic process to lower jaw.

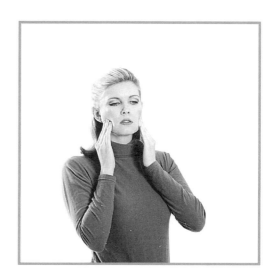

Obliquus Capitis Inferior

obliquus = oblique, slanting, muscle fibers running diagonally to midline of body; capitis = of the head; inferior = lower

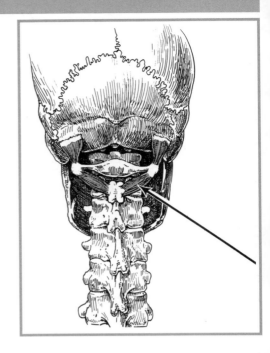

Muscle Facts
Origin:
The apex of the spinous process of the axis (C2).

Insertion:
The inferior and dorsal part of the transverse process of the atlas (C1).

Action:
Unilaterally, rotates the atlas, turning the face toward the same side. Bilaterally, extend the neck backwards.

Method of Testing
Muscle Test:
Use a surrogate muscle.

Circuit Localize:
Between the spinous process of the axis and the transverse process of the atlas.

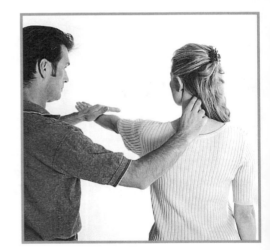

Biokinetic Exercise
Turn your face far to the left and then upwards. Place right hand on top of head and rock head backwards slightly. Use left hand to press right side of chin up and to the left.

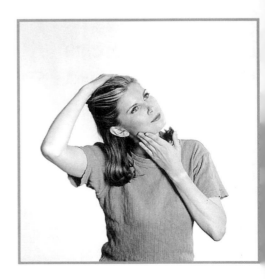

Obliquus Capitis Superior

obliquus = oblique, slanting, muscle fibers running diagonally to midline of body; capitis = of the head; superior = upper

Muscle Facts

Origin:
The superior surface of the transverse process of the atlas.

Insertion:
Between the superior and inferior nuchal lines of the occipital bone.

Action:
Extension and lateral flexion of head at neck.

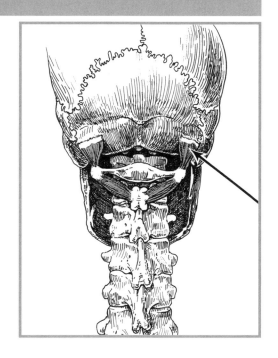

Method of Testing

Muscle Test:
Use a surrogate muscle.

Circuit Localize:
Between the transverse process of the atlas and the occipital bone.

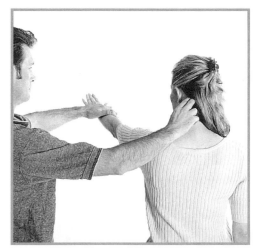

Biokinetic Exercise

Sit upright. Turn head 20° to the right. Place hand under the chin and gently tilt head backwards.

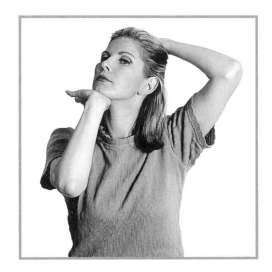

Opponens Digiti Minimi

opponens = opposing; digit = finger; minimis = smallest

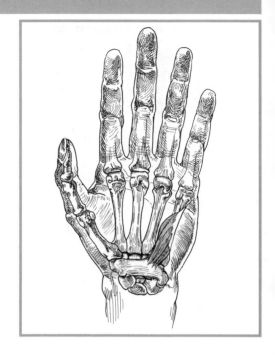

Muscle Facts

Origin:
Convex surface of the hamate bone and the adjoining portion of the transverse carpal ligament.

Insertion:
Entire length of ulnar border of metacarpal bone of the little finger.

Action:
Flexes and slightly laterally rotates the fifth finger. Helps to cup the palm of the hand.

Method of Testing

Muscle Test:
Stabilize the hand, especially the thumb side. The little finger is flexed and turned slightly toward the thumb. Pressure is on the base of the little finger to straighten it.

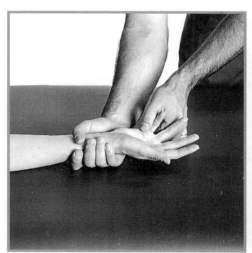

Circuit Localize:
Middle of the medial palm in line with the little finger.

Biokinetic Exercise

Place bent elbow on thigh. Flex wrist fully so that finger tips are close to the biceps. Support back of wrist with right hand. With thumb on metacarpophalangeal joint of little finger push down towards outer side of elbow joint.

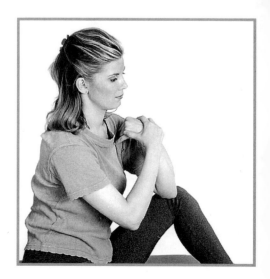

Opponens Pollicis

opponens = opposing muscle; pollicis = of the thumb

Muscle Facts

Origin:
Flexor retinaculum and tubercle on trapezium bone.

Insertion:
Entire length of first metacarpal bone on the radial side.

Action:
Opposition, which is a partial medial rotation of the metacarpal of the thumb. By its use the tip of the thumb can be made to meet the tips of the four fingers in turn.

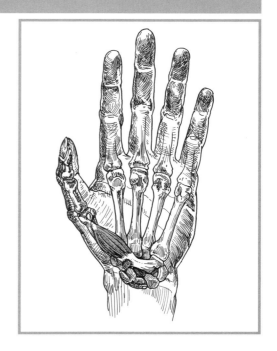

Method of Testing

Muscle Test:
Have the person being tested touch the tip of the thumb to the tip of the little finger, making a ring. Keep the other fingers fully extended and straight as possible. Place a finger from each hand inside this ring and attempt to pull the thumb and little finger apart. If the muscles lock after coming apart just a bit, they may be considered strong. This also evaluates the opponens minimi digiti connecting to the fifth metacarpal.

Circuit Localize:
Into fleshy pad of hand.

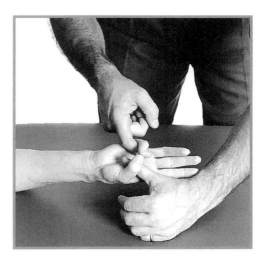

Biokinetic Exercise

Press the dorsal side of the thumb toward the medial palmar side of the wrist. Hold.

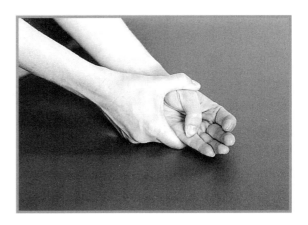

Palmaris Longus

palma = palm; longus = long

Muscle Facts
This muscle is absent in about 13% of individuals.

Origin:
Common flexor tendon from medial epicondyle of humerus.

Insertion:
Flexor retinaculum and palmar aponeurosis.

Action:
Flexes hand at the wrist.

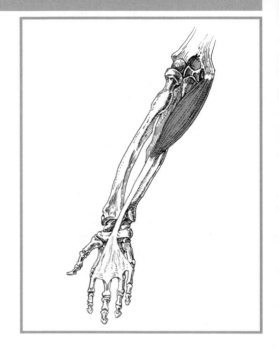

Method of Testing
Muscle Test:
Flex wrist up, with forearm stabilized on table. Test by trying to pull wrist out, as if to touch back of hand to table.

Circuit Localize:
Medial side anterior forearm, just distal of the elbow joint.

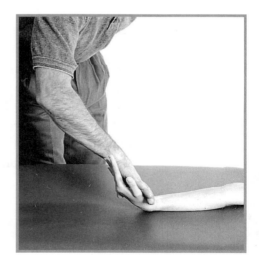

Biokinetic Exercise
1. In a sitting position, flex your arm and rest your elbow on your hip.
2. Turn your palm down, curl your fingers.
3. Press the back of your hand towards the inside of your elbow.

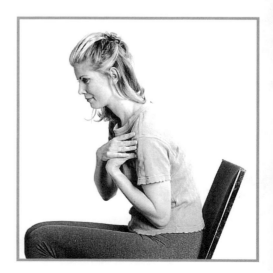

Pectineus

pecten = comb

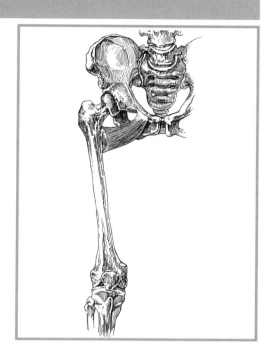

Muscle Facts

Origin:
A space about an inch wide on the front of the pubes, just below the rim of the pelvic basin between the iliopectineal eminence and the tubercle of the pubis.

Insertion:
Pectineal line of femur, from lesser trochanter to linea aspera.

Action:
The pectineus is a prime mover for hip joint flexion and adduction. It is a weak assistant for medial rotation.

Method of Testing

Muscle Test:
With client lying on back place leg 45° out to the side. Turn foot out 30°. Pressure is against the lower leg to take it further to the side.

Circuit Localize:
In the fold between the upper thigh and the lower abdomen.

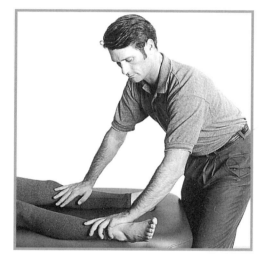

Biokinetic Exercise

1. Stand, place your left foot to the right of the right foot.
2. Keep your legs straight and bend forward.

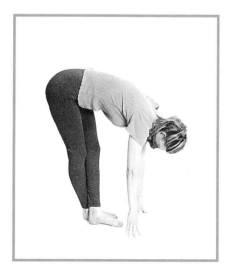

Pectoralis Major Clavicular

pectoralis = of the chest or breast; major = greater; clavicular = of the collar bone

Muscle Facts
Origin:
Anterior surface of the medial half of the clavicle.

Insertion:
By a flat tendon about three inches wide into the ridge that forms the outer border of the intertubercular groove of the humerus, extending from just below the tuberosities nearly down to the insertion of the deltoid.

Action:
Flexion, adduction, horizontal flexion and medial rotation of the humerus at the shoulder.

Method of Testing
Muscle Test:
The client holds the arm straight, directed forward with the arm in medial rotation so that thumb points toward the feet. Stabilizing the opposite shoulder, pressure is at the distal end of the forearm to push it out and slightly down, following the direction of the fibers.

Circuit Localize:
One thumb width below the middle portion of the clavicle.

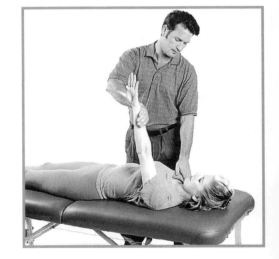

Biokinetic Exercise
For left side:
1. Cross your left arm in front of you over to your right side, turn the palm down and then keep turning it until back of the elbow faces forward.
2. With your right hand grasp your left arm and pull it straight across toward your opposite shoulder. Rest

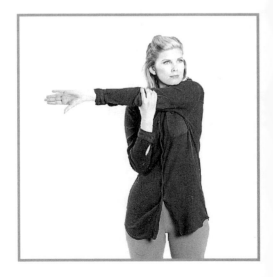

Pectoralis Major Sternal

pectoralis = of the chest or breast; major = greater; sternal = of the breast bone

Muscle Facts

Origin:
Half of breadth of anterior surface of sternum as far as sixth or seventh rib, cartilages of first six or seven ribs.

Insertion:
By a flat tendon about three inches wide into the ridge that forms the outer border of the intertubercular groove of the humerus, extending from just below the tuberosities nearly down to the insertion of the deltoid.

Action:
A prime mover for extension and adduction. Both sternal and clavicular portions of the pectoralis major muscle assist in medial rotation and horizontal flexion.

Method of Testing

Muscle Test:
The client holds their arm straight, directed forwards with the arm in medial rotation so the thumb points toward the feet. Pressure is at the distal end of the forearm to push it out and up following the direction of the fibers. Stabilize the opposite shoulder or hip.

Circuit Localize:
Three thumb widths above the nipple.

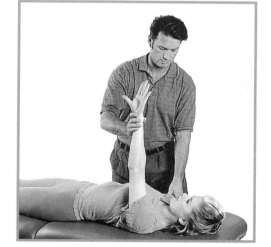

Biokinetic Exercise

1. Cross your left arm in front of you over to your right side, turn the palm down and then keep turning it until it faces forwards.
2. With your right hand grasp your left wrist (or elbow) and pull it down to the right across the lower ribs. Rest.

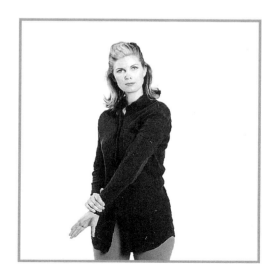

Pectoralis Minor

pectoralis = of the chest or breast; minor = lesser

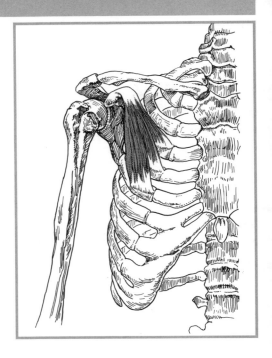

Muscle Facts
Origin:
The anterior surfaces of the third, fourth, and fifth ribs near the costal cartilages. Some people have part of this muscle group originating on the second rib.

Insertion:
The coracoid process of the scapula.

Action:
Pulls the coracoid process inwards, forwards and downwards; rotates shoulder joint anteriorly.
Reversed Origin-Insertion Action: When the scapula is fixed, it aids in rib elevation in forced inspiration.

Method of Testing
Muscle Test:
Person is supine and holds shoulder up off the table drawing it forwards, downwards and inwards. Pressure is to move the shoulder upwards and backwards towards the table.

Circuit Localize:
In line, between the coracoid process of the scapula and the costal cartilages of the third, fourth, and fifth ribs.

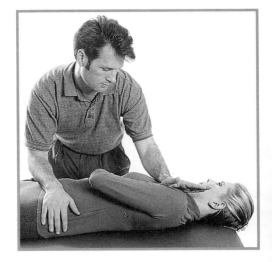

Biokinetic Exercise
For left side:
1. Sitting on the edge of a chair, bring your right foot up near your left knee and grasp it with your left hand.
2. Pull your right foot down and to the right, holding on to it with your left hand while bending your left shoulder down and to the right.
3. Drop your head forwards. Rest while breathing deeply.

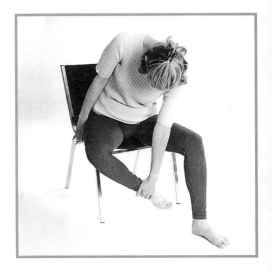

Peroneus Tertius

perone = fibula; tertius = third

Muscle Facts

Origin:
Distal third of the anterior surface of the fibula, interosseous membrane and adjacent intermuscular septum.

Insertion:
Dorsal surface of the base of the fifth metatarsal.

Action:
Dorsiflexes and everts the foot

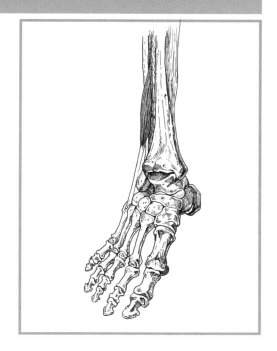

Method of Testing

Muscle Test:
Begin with the foot flexed back and out to the side (dorsal flexion and eversion) with the toes straight or curled down. Stabilize the back of the lower leg just above the ankle so it does not move during the test. Placing the palm on the top outside of the foot just behind the toes, press down and in toward the midline. Make sure client does not bend the toes back and so bringing other muscles into the test.

Circuit Localize:
Touch on the lateral side of the lower leg one palm width above and just forward of the lateral malleolus.

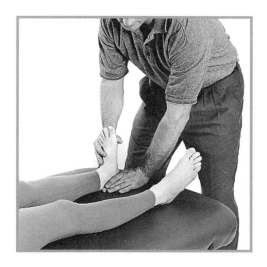

Biokinetic Exercise

1. Sit on the floor with your knees up.
2. Grasp the lateral side of the foot near the little toe; pull upwards toward the outside of the knees.

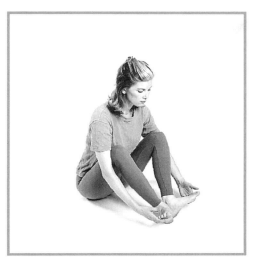

Piriformis

pirum = pear; forma = shape

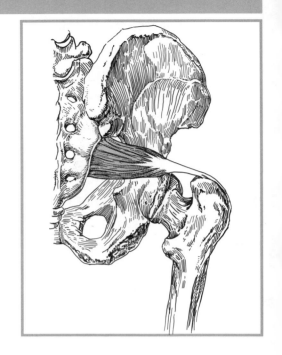

Muscle Facts

Origin:
Anterior surface of sacrum between and lateral to anterior sacral foramina; margin of the greater sciatic foramen; anterior surface of sacrotuberous ligament.

Insertion:
Superior border of greater trochanter of femur.

Action:
Rotates thigh laterally and abducts the flexed thigh at the hip.

Method of Testing

Muscle Test:
Client lies face up. The knee and hip are bent at right angles and the foot brought across the opposite leg as far as possible. Pressure is against the inside of the ankle to bring the foot out to the side while stabilizing the knee.

Circuit Localize:
Mid-upper portion of buttocks between greater trochanter of femur and midline of body.

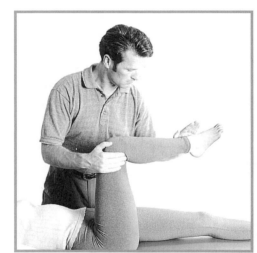

Biokinetic Exercise

Lie on your stomach and put your knees way out to the sides, placing the soles of your feet together near the groin. If you can't keep your hips down, don't strain — relax with your hips up a few inches.

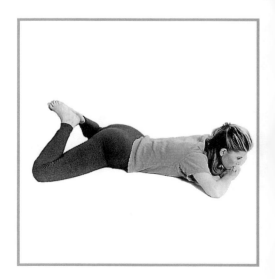

Plantar Interossi

plantar = sole of the foot; interossei = between the bones

Muscle Facts
Origin:
These three plantar interossei arise from the bases and medial plantar surfaces of the third, fourth and fifth metatarsal bones.

Insertion:
The medial sides of the proximal phalanges of the same toes and the tendons of the extensor digitorum longus.

Action:
Adducts the third, fourth and fifth toes toward the second toe. Flex the proximal and extend the distal phalanges of the third, fourth and fifth toes.

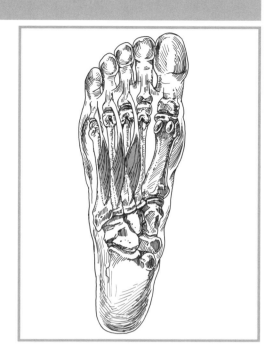

Method of Testing
Muscle Test:
Use a surrogate muscle.

Circuit Localize:
On the plantar surface of the foot on the medial sides of the third, fourth and fifth metatarsals.

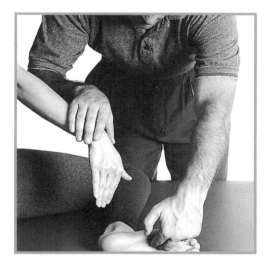

Biokinetic Exercise
For left side:
1. With the right thumb, compress the middle of the sole of the left foot toward the third toe.
2. At the same time, with the left hand press the base of the third toe both medially and towards the heel. Rest.
3. Repeat for the fourth and fifth toes.

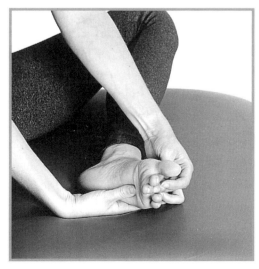

Popliteus

poples = the ham of the knee

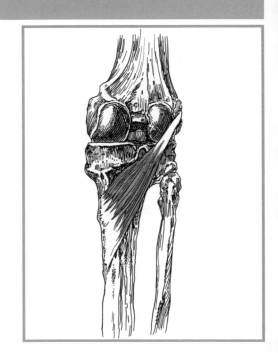

Muscle Facts
Origin:
Primarily, the deep depression on the outer side of the external condyle of the femur; also the postero-medial aspect of the head of the fibula, and the posterior horn of the lateral meniscus.

Insertion: Medial posterior side of tibia, superior to the origin of the soleus.

Action:
Inward rotation of the tibia, or, when the tibia is fixed during weight bearing, outward rotation of the femur on the tibia. Withdraws the meniscus during flexion, and provides rotatory stability to the femur on the tibia. Brings the knee out of the position of full extension. Helps with posterior stability of the knee.

Method of Testing
Muscle Test:
Client lies face down. Bend the knee to 90° and rotate the tibia medially. With the ankle bent at 90°, pressure is against the inside of the foot, using it as a lever to rotate the tibia laterally.

Circuit Localize:
Just below the knee on the posterior part of the upper calf.

Biokinetic Exercise
1. Sit on the floor with your legs folded back and to the sides, point your toes in.
2. Place your hands on your heels and press them laterally and towards your knees.
3. Raise yourself off the floor by pressing your knees outward. Rest.

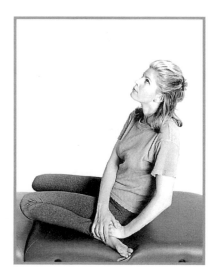

Pronator Quadratus

pronator = muscle that turns the palm downward or posteriorly; quadratus = square

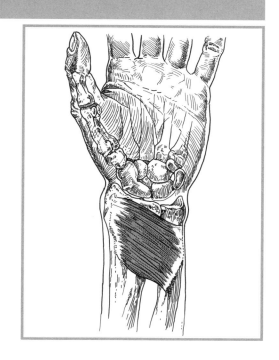

Muscle Facts
Origin:
Distal quarter of the anterior surface of the ulna.

Insertion:
Distal quarter of the anterior surface of the radius.

Action:
Works with the pronator teres muscle to pronate the forearm (turns the hand palm down, thumb in), regardless of the angle of the elbow joint. Helps stabilize the carpal tunnel at the wrist.

Method of Testing
Muscle Test:
Hold elbow to side with forearm flexed to at least 140° (to put pronator teres at a disadvantage), palm facing forwards away from body. Pressure is at the wrist to turn the thumb up and out.

Circuit Localize:
One thumb above anterior wrist joint, obliquely on forearm.

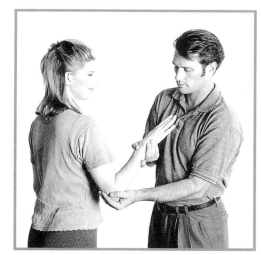

Biokinetic Exercise
1. Grasp the anterior surface of your left wrist with your right hand, with your right fingers on the thumb side and your palm on the little finger side of the wrist.
2. Squeeze the fingers of your right hand towards the right palm.

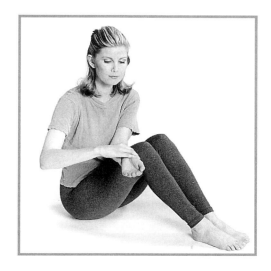

Pronator Teres

pronator = muscle that turns palm downward or posteriorly; teres = round, smooth

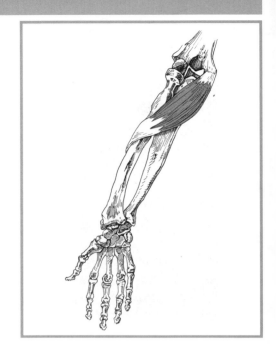

Muscle Facts
Origin:
Humeral Head: Medial epicondyle of humerus.
Ulnar Head: Medial side of coronoid process of ulna (joins humeral head at acute angle).

Insertion:
Middle one-third of lateral surface of radius.

Action:
Turns palm down (pronates it) by rotating the radius upon the ulna. Helps flex forearm at the elbow.

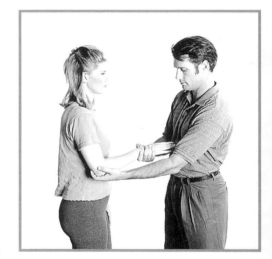

Method of Testing
Muscle Test:
Hold elbow to side with forearm flexed 90° and rotated medially so that the palm is down. Support elbow. Pressure is at wrist to rotate palm up and out.

Circuit Localize:
Just below anterior elbow joint, on forearm.

Biokinetic Exercise
1. Flex your arm 120°, point your fingers forward and palm down.
2. Grasp your left hand with your right hand and forcibly twist it to the left (outwards), pressing your left hand toward your left elbow.

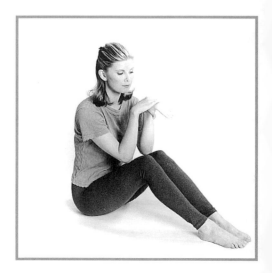

Psoas Major

psoa = muscles of the loins

Muscle Facts

Origin:
Transverse processes of all lumbar vertebrae. Sides of bodies of last thoracic and all lumbar vertebrae and corresponding lateral surfaces of the intervertebral discs.

Insertion:
Lesser trochanter of the femur.

Action:
Flexes and rotates thigh laterally.
Reversed Origin - Insertion Action: The psoas paradox: When the thigh is kept stationary, generally when the body is in supine lying position, the psoas and iliacus muscles flex the hip joint, pulling on the lumbar vertebrae in anterior and inferior direction, as in sit-ups.

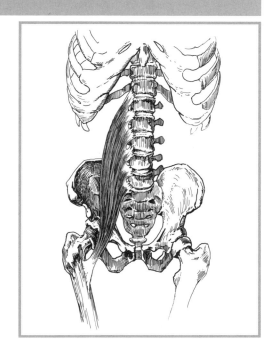

Method of Testing

Muscle Test:
Raise the leg to 45° and slightly out to the side with the foot rotated out. With the opposite hip stabilized, pressure is against the inside of the ankle, pulling or pushing the leg back and slightly out.

Circuit Localize:
Just above fold, between upper thigh and lower abdomen.

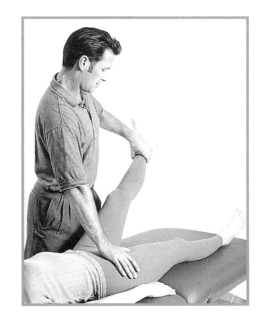

Biokinetic Exercise

Lying on your back, bring your left knee up toward your right shoulder. Grasp behind your left thigh and pull it toward your abdomen. Rest.

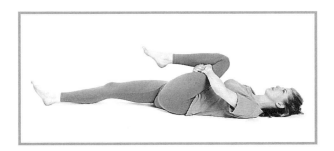

Pterygoid Lateral – external pterygoid

*pterygoid = like a wing – relates to pterygoid plate of sphenoid;
lateral = farther from midline*

Muscle Facts
Origin:
Superior Head: Inferior part of lateral surface of great wing of sphenoid.
Inferior Head: Lateral surface of lateral pterygoid plate.

Insertion:
Anterior aspect of neck of condyle of mandible; anterior margin of articular disk of temporomandibular articulation.

Action:
Bilaterally, act to protract mandible (pull jaw forward), open jaw. Unilaterally, moves mandible to opposite side, thus left pterygoid lateral pulls the mandible towards the right and the right muscle pulls the right mandible towards the left, as in rotary chewing.

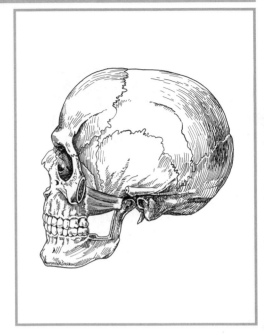

Method of Testing
Muscle Test:
Use a surrogate muscle for this muscle test.

Circuit Localize:
Between upper neck of mandible and sphenoid bone.

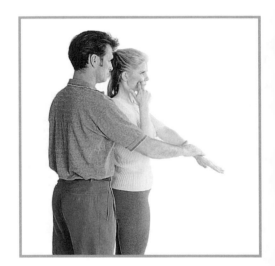

Biokinetic Exercise
Drop the jaw. Forcibly pull ramus of jaw forward and up. Rest.

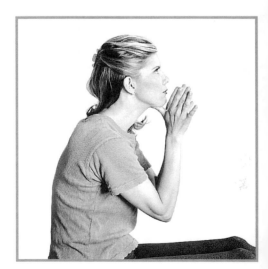

Pterygoid Medial – internal pterygoid

pterygoid = like a wing – relates to pterygoid plate of sphenoid; medial = closer to midline

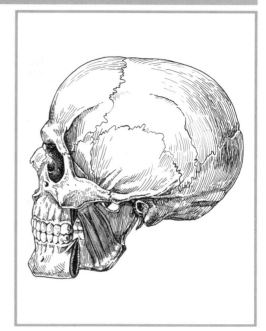

Muscle Facts

Origin:
Medial surface of lateral pterygoid plate of sphenoid. Pyramidal process of palatine bone.

Insertion:
Inferior and posterior parts of medial surface of ramus and angle of mandible.

Action:
Elevates and pulls mandible forwards. Moves mandible from side-to-side. The left pterygoid medial pulls to the right, the right pterygoid medial pulls to the left.

Method of Testing

Muscle Test:
Use a surrogate muscle for this muscle test.

Circuit Localize:
Inside the mouth, pointing directly back, behind upper molars.

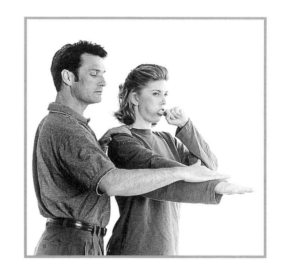

Biokinetic Exercise

1. Open your mouth wide and touch the muscle going between the upper and lower jaw.
2. Relax the jaw (without closing it) and gently and firmly massage the muscle upwards.

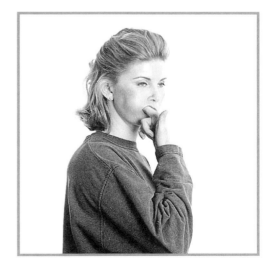

Pyramidalis

pyramis = pyramid

Muscle Facts

Origin:
Anterior aspect of the symphysis pubis and pubic bone.

Insertion:
Into the linea alba, midway between the pubic bone and the navel.

Action:
Compresses the abdomen, supports abdominal organs and tenses the linea alba.

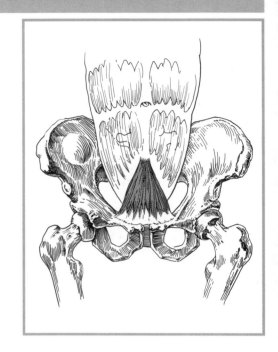

Method of Testing

Muscle Test:
Client sits with legs straight and trunk bent forward to 110° and the left shoulder rotated 23° forwards. The arms are crossed with hands on opposite shoulders. Practitioner braces on left thigh. Pressure is on the left upper chest to push straight back.

Circuit Localize:
On midline, one thumb width above top of pubic bone.

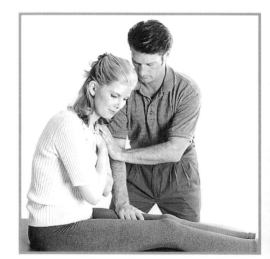

Biokinetic Exercise

Sitting on the floor, bend forward and press down on abdominal muscles below your navel.

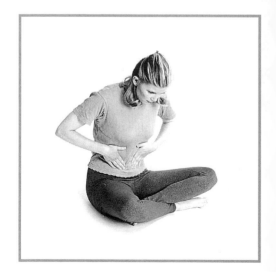

Quadratus Lumborum

quadratus = square; lumbus = loin

Muscle Facts

Origin:
Iliolumbar ligament, posterior part of the iliac crest.

Insertion:
Medial half of inferior border of last rib and transverse processes of the upper four lumbar vertebrae.

Action:
Lateral flexion of lumbar vertebral column. When both of these muscles act together, they depress the last ribs and assist in holding them down when the diaphragm contracts.

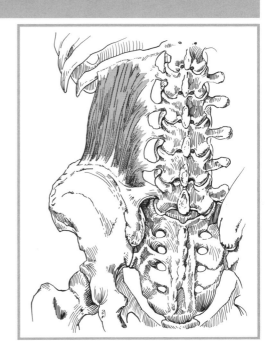

Method of Testing

Muscle Test:
Client lies face up and holds on to sides of table. Take both legs out to one side, stabilize at the opposite hip. Pressure is at the outside of the ankle to press both legs toward the midline.

Circuit Localize:
In line between the iliac crest and the lumbar vertebrae.

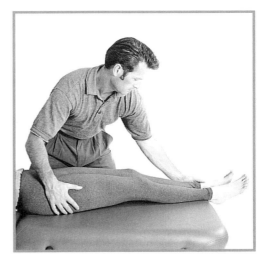

Biokinetic Exercise

For Left Side:
1. Stand with your feet about two feet apart. Put your left hand on your upper left hip and push it to the right and upwards.
2. Bend far to the left, with your left shoulder down and your right shoulder up and slightly back. Rest.

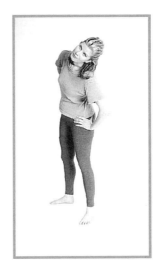

Rectus Abdominis

rectus = erect, straight up; abdominis = of the belly or the abdomen

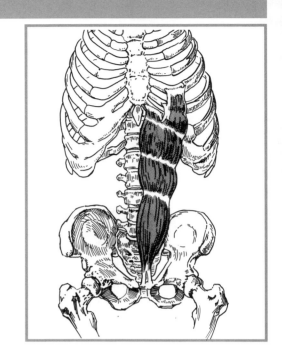

Muscle Facts

Origin:
Pubic crest and symphysis pubis.

Insertion:
The costal cartilages of the fifth through seventh ribs and the side of the xiphoid process.

Action:
Flexes vertebral column at lumbar spine and compresses abdomen. Lateral flexion of trunk. In standing position, gives anterior support to abdominal organs and lumbar spine. With aid of gluteus maximus and hamstrings keeps pelvis from going into anterior tilt.

Method of Testing

Muscle Test:
Person being tested sits with knees bent and together, hands on the opposite shoulders, leaning back, chin up. Pressure is against the wrists where they cross, to push backwards. Stabilize the thighs by placing a forearm above the knees as you test. Person testing should cross arms for better leverage.

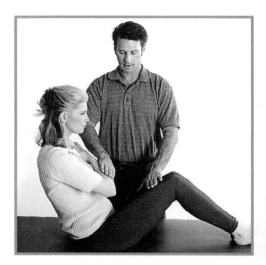

Circuit Localize:
Rectus abdominis is divided into four or five segments bounded by tendinous intersections. Most anatomists show one segment below the navel, biokinesiology recognizes two.

Biokinetic Exercise

For muscle segments below the navel: Sit on the floor and lean forward pressing your abdominal muscles down from an area just above your navel; **or** clasp your hands behind you and sag your chest forward and down.

For muscle segments above the navel: Sit on the floor and bend forwards. Place your hands on your rectus abdominis muscles just inferior to your navel and pull up firmly. Rest while breathing deeply.

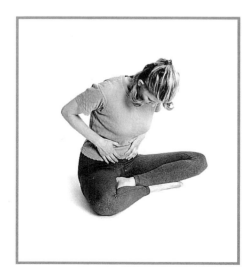

Rectus Capitis Anterior

rectus = straight; capitis = of the head; anterior = front

Muscle Facts

Origin:
Anterior surface of the lateral mass of the atlas and the root of its transverse process.

Insertion:
The inferior surface of the basilar part of the occipital bone anterior to the occipital condyle and foramen magnum (hole for spinal cord).

Action:
Aids in flexion of the head at the neck.

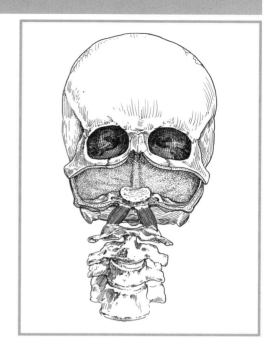

Method of Testing

Muscle Test:
Use a surrogate muscle.

Circuit Localize:
Pointing up and in towards the front of the atlas from just posterior and superior to the ramus of the jaw on the side of the neck.

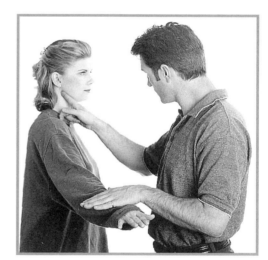

Biokinetic Exercise

For Left Side:
1. Flex head forwards.
2. Drop left ear down towards left shoulder.
3. Use left hand to press crown of head down towards left shoulder. Rest.

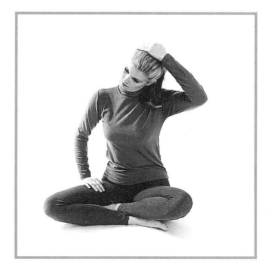

89

Rectus Capitis Lateralis

rectus = straight; capitis = of the head; lateralis = side

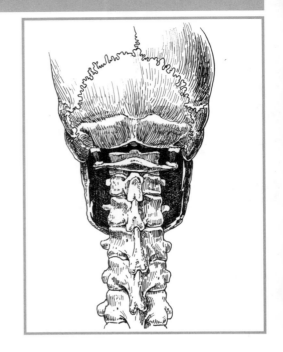

Muscle Facts
Origin:
Superior surface of the transverse process of the atlas (C1).

Insertion:
Inferior surface of the jugular process of the occipital bone.

Action:
Assists in lateral flexion of the head on the neck.

Method of Testing
Muscle Test:
Use a surrogate muscle.

Circuit Localize:
Deep, immediately above outer part of transverse process of atlas.

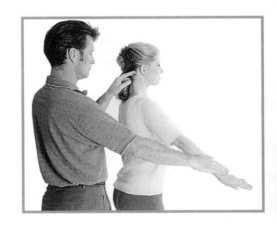

Biokinetic Exercise
1. Tilt your head fully back looking up behind you. Press the top of your head towards your chest and your chin up as high as you can push it. Rest.
2. Tilt your face 45° to the left and resume the same pressures. Rest.

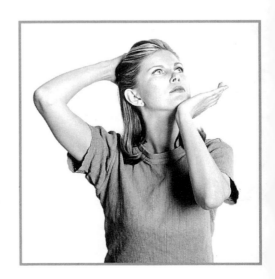

Rectus Capitis Posterior Major

rectus = straight; capitis = of the head; posterior = back; major = greater

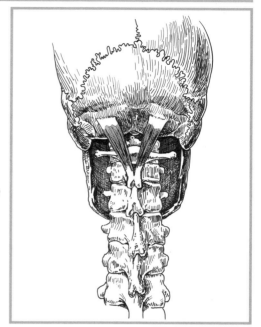

Muscle Facts

Origin:
The spinous process of the axis (C2).

Insertion:
The lateral part of the inferior nuchal line of the occipital bone (outside of rectus capitis posterior minor) and the surface of the bone immediately inferior to the line.

Action:
Extends the head and rotates it to the same side.

Method of Testing

Muscle Test:
Use a surrogate muscle for this muscle test.

Circuit Localize:
One thumb lateral of the midline of the spine, press deep just below the occipital bone.

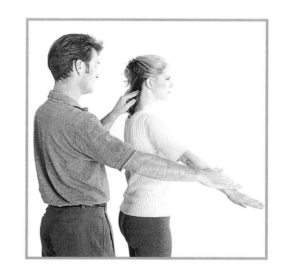

Biokinetic Exercise

1. With your right hand, press your left chin far to the right and upwards.
2. With your left hand pull superior posterior part of your head down and forward towards your Adam's apple, arching back slightly. Rest.

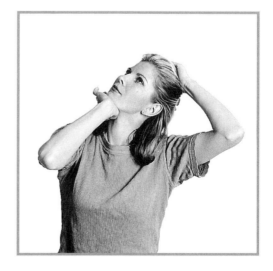

Rectus Capitis Posterior Minor

rectus = straight; capitis = of the head; posterior = back; minor = lesser

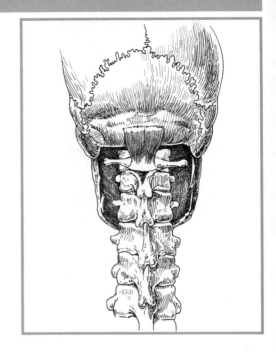

Muscle Facts

Origin:
The tubercle on the posterior arch of the atlas.

Insertion:
The medial part of the inferior nuchal line of the occipital bone.

Action:
Extends the head at the neck.

Method of Testing

Muscle Test:
Use a surrogate muscle.

Circuit Localize:
Half a thumb lateral of the midline of the spine, press deep just below the occipital bone.

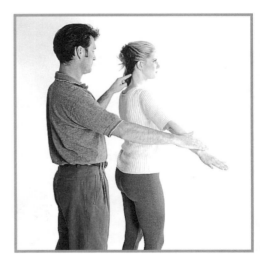

Biokinetic Exercise

Press the chin up, the back of the head down and forward.

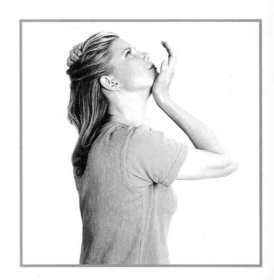

Rectus Femoris

rectus = straight; femoris = of the thigh

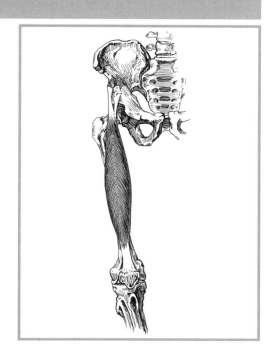

Muscle Facts
1 of the 4 muscles of the Quadriceps

Origin:
Straight Head: Anterior inferior spine of ilium.
Reflected Head: Groove on upper brim of the acetabulum.

Insertion:
Proximal border of patella and through the patellar ligament into tibial tuberosity.

Action:
Extends the leg at the knee, flexes thigh at hip joint.
Reversed Origin – Insertion Action: Flexes the pelvis on the femur and gives anterior stabilization to the pelvis.

Method of Testing
Muscle Test:
Client supine, raise femur 70°, lower leg is horizontal. Press raised knee to extend leg back to table.

Circuit Localize:
In the middle of the midline of the anterior thigh.

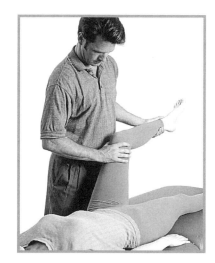

Biokinetic Exercise
1. Stand with your feet about one-and-one-half feet apart pointing your feet forward.
2. Bend forwards from the hips until your body is horizontal.
3. Grasp your knee caps and pull them upwards keeping your knees locked backwards.

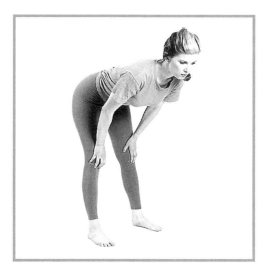

Rhomboid Major

rhomboides = rhomboid or diamond-shaped; major = greater

Muscle Facts

Origin:
Spinous processes of second to fifth thoracic vertebrae.

Insertion:
Medial border of scapula from spine to inferior angle.

Action:
Adducts lower angle of scapula without adducting the upper angle at all. Assist in rotating the glenoid cavity downwards.

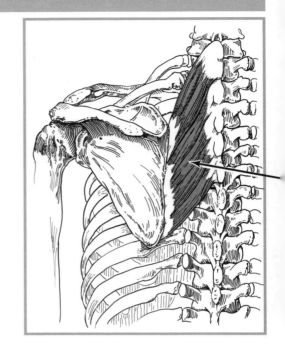

Method of Testing

Muscle Test:
With the elbow bent and held against the side, stabilize the shoulder. Pressure is against the inside of the upper arm to pull it away from the side.

Circuit Localize:
Midway between T2-T5 and medial border of scapula.

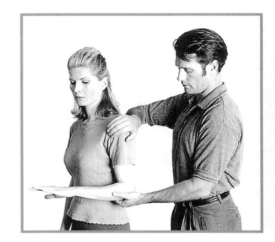

Biokinetic Exercise

1. Get on your hands and knees and place your hands about three or four feet apart (depending on your size) and straight out from your shoulders keeping arms straight.
2. Attempt to sag down in the area between your shoulder blades. This causes a winging back of your shoulder blades and a compression of them towards your spine. Rest in this position breathing deeply.

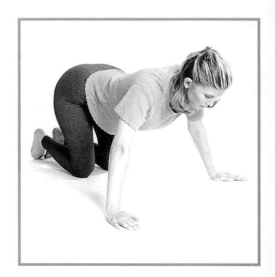

Rhomboid Minor

rhomboides = rhomboid or diamond-shaped; minor = lesser

Muscle Facts

Origin:
Inferior part of ligamentum nuchae, spinous processes of seventh cervical and first thoracic vertebrae.

Insertion:
Medial border of scapula at the root of the spine of the scapula.

Action:
Adducts scapula. Retracts and elevates the scapula. Assists in rotating the inferior angle of the scapula medially.

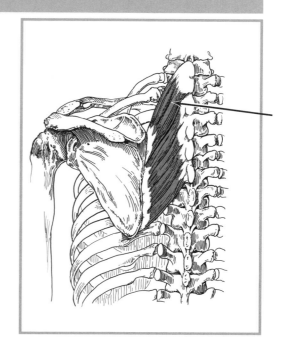

Method of Testing

Muscle Test:
Place hand on hip, thumb forward and palm on gluteal area, and elbow drawn back. Stabilize the shoulder. Apply pressure on the back of the elbow to push it anteriorly (thereby medially rotating the humerus).

Circuit Localize:
Lateral and inferior to C7 and T1 spinous processes.

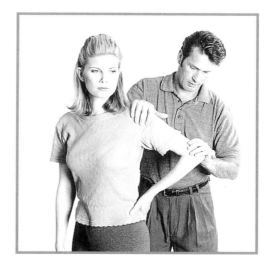

Biokinetic Exercise

1. Get down on your hands and knees, placing your hands about three feet apart and about one foot in front of your shoulders.
2. Drop your head and chest while permitting your shoulder blades to come together. The area between your shoulder blades must sag down toward the floor.

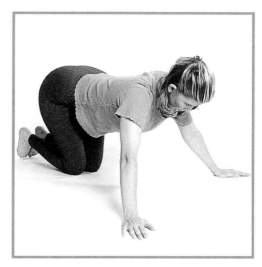

Rotatores Brevis

rotatores = rotators; brevis = short

Muscle Facts
A series of pairs of small muscles extending from the sacrum to the axis.

Origin:
Transverse processes of the vertebrae.

Insertion:
Bases of the spinous processes of the vertebra next above.

Action:
Acting unilaterally, rotation of the spine to the opposite side. Acting bilaterally, extension of the spine.

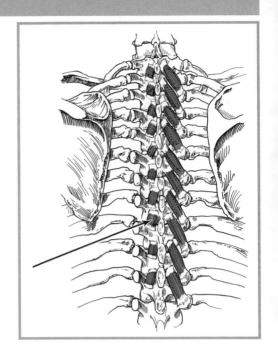

Method of Testing
Muscle Test:
Use a surrogate muscle.

Circuit Localize:
Posteriorily into the spine, midway between the spinous process of one vertebra and the transverse process of the vertebra immediately below it.

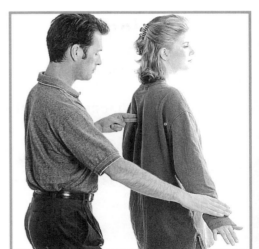

Biokinetic Exercise
For example, rotator brevis T8:
1. Place right thumb or fingers on the right side of spinous process of T8.
2. Arch left shoulder back, twisting slightly to the left. Left hand can be placed on hip for support, if needed. Rest.

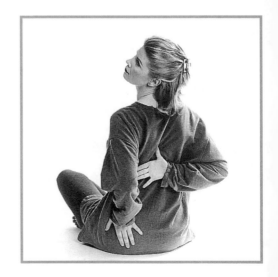

Rotatores Longus

rotatores = rotators; longus = long

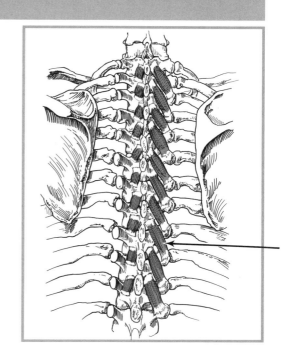

Muscle Facts
A series of pairs of small muscles extending from the sacrum to the axis.

Origin:
Transverse processes of the vertebrae.

Insertion:
Bases of the spinous processes of the vertebra two above its origin.

Action:
Acting unilaterally, rotation of the spine to the opposite side, flexion to the side. Acting bilaterally, extension and hyperextension of the spine.

Method of Testing

Muscle Test:
Use a surrogate muscle for this muscle test.

Circuit Localize:
Posteriorly into the spine, midway between the transverse process of one vertebra and the spinousprocess of the second vertebra above it.

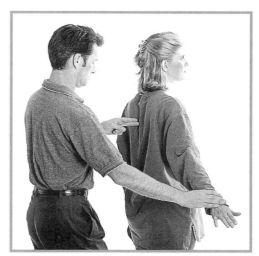

Biokinetic Exercise
1. Sit on the floor with your legs folded behind you and to the sides.
2. Grasp your right foot behind you with your left hand and pull your left shoulder back towards your right side. Rest.
3. While arching back, you could press the transverse process of a specific vertebra up and to the right with your right hand. Rest.

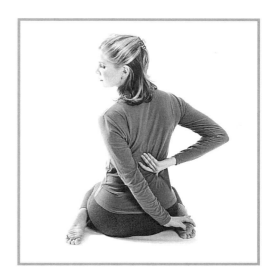

Sartorius

sartor = tailor; refers to cross-legged position of tailors

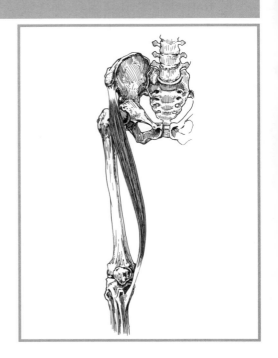

Muscle Facts

Origin:
The anterior superior iliac spine and the upper half of the iliac notch.

Insertion:
Anteromedial surface of tibial bone posterior to the tuberosity.

Action:
Directly assists in flexion, abduction, and lateral rotation of the thigh at the hip joint. In most individuals sartorius is a knee flexor, but in some it serves as a knee extensor.
Reversed Origin – Insertion Action: When femur and knee are fixed, flexes the pelvis on the hip and gives anterior stabilization to the pelvis.

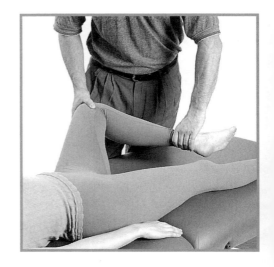

Method of Testing

Muscle Test:
Flex the hip and the knee with abduction of the hip so the knee is rotated laterally and the foot over the opposite knee. Place one hand on the outside of the knee and push it toward adduction as you attempt to straighten the leg.

Circuit Localize:
One palm above anterior knee and three thumbwidths medial of the vertical midline of the thigh.

Biokinetic Exercise

1. Sit on floor in a semi-tailor fashion, crossing your ankles, your knees out 45° and your feet about one foot from your groin.
2. Grasp the upper part of the lower legs and lean back.

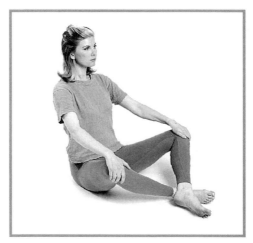

Semimembranosus

semi = half; membran = membrane

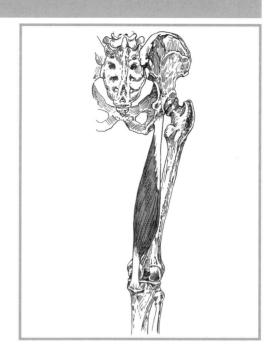

Muscle Facts
1 of the 3 muscles making up the Hamstrings

Origin:
Upper and lateral aspect of ischial tuberosity.

Insertion:
Horizontal groove on posterior medial aspect of medial condyle of tibia.

Action:
Extends, adducts and medially rotates the thigh at the hip. Flexes and medially rotates the leg at the knee.

Method of Testing
Muscle Test:
Client prone, raise the lower leg 90° and rotate it medially 15°. Put support pressure in the middle of the hamstrings to prevent cramping. Pressure is against the back of the achilles tendon to straighten the leg.

Circuit Localize:
On the posterior medial side of the thigh.

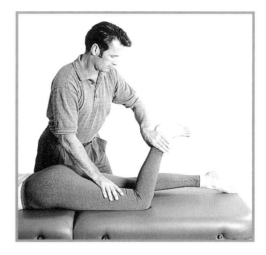

Biokinetic Exercise
1. Kneel upright, place the left knee about one foot behind the right knee, keep your legs together.
2. Pull the left foot up towards your left buttocks with your right hand and arch back.
3. Place most of your weight on your left knee. Rest.

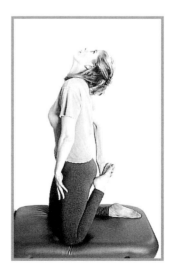

Semitendinosus

semi = half; tendo = tendon

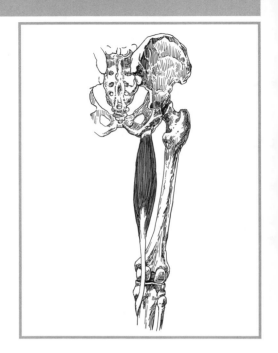

Muscle Facts
1 of the 3 muscles making up the Hamstrings

Origin:
Distal and medial impression on ischial tuberosity with tendon of the long head of the biceps femoris.

Insertion:
Anteromedial surface of tibia at proximal end of shaft just below the condyle.

Action:
Extends, adducts and medially rotates the thigh at the hip. Flexes and medially rotates the leg at the knee.

Method of Testing
Muscle Test:
Client prone, flexes the lower leg 90°. Put support pressure in the middle of the thigh to prevent cramping. Pressure is against the back of the achilles tendon to straighten the leg.

Circuit Localize:

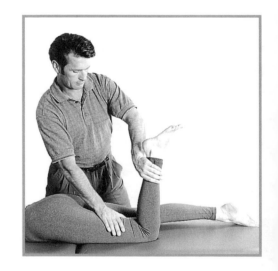

Biokinetic Exercise
1. Kneel, place your left knee back eight inches from your right knee.
2. Pull your left lower leg up with your left hand.
3. Twist the left leg out 20°, placing your weight on your left leg.
4. Arch back, hold for 30 seconds.

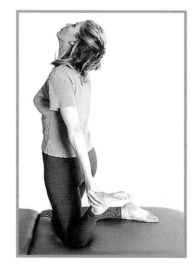

Serratus Anterior

serratus = serrated; anterior = front

Muscle Facts

Origin:
The outer surfaces and superior borders of upper eight or nine ribs at the side of the chest.

Insertion:
The anterior surface of the medial border of the scapula, from the superior to the inferior angle.

Action:
The prime mover for abduction and upward rotation of the scapula. Stabilizes vertebral border of scapula to thoracic cage along with rhomboids and middle trapezius.

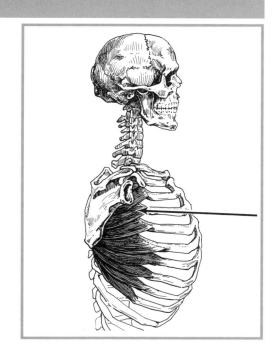

Method of Testing

Muscle Test:
Hold the arm in front and slightly out to the side, thumb up and level with the top of the head. Pressure is against the forearm to push it toward the feet. The facilitator's other hand contacts the bottom outside border of the scapula to feel for any movement backwards or toward the spine. Any movement detected here or in the arm indicates that the muscle is not 100%.

Circuit Localize:
Just under armpit and down side of chest.

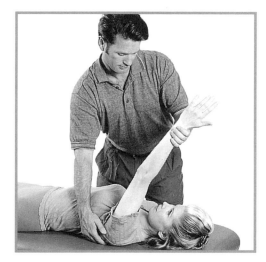

Biokinetic Exercise

1. Reach under your left arm pit and grasp your shoulder blade with your right hand.
2. Pull the shoulder blade forwards and up while relaxing the left shoulder.

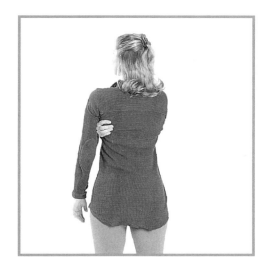

Serratus Anterior #5 Tendon

serratus = serrated; anterior = front; #5 = fifth portion of muscle group according to Biokinesiology

Tendon Facts
Origin:
Outer surface and upper border of the fourth rib.

Insertion:
Upper vertebral border of scapula.

Action:
Draws scapula forward.

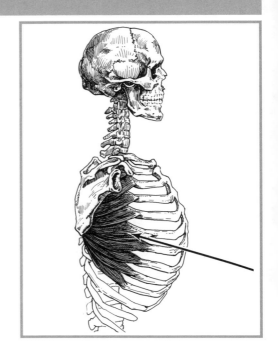

Method of Testing
Muscle Test:
Left arm horizontal, thumb up, 45° lateral of forward. Stabilize shoulder. Attempt to push arm towards feet.

Circuit Localize:
Upper border of fourth rib under armpit.

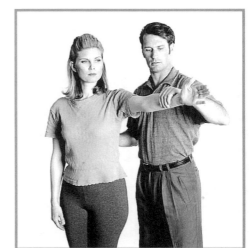

Biokinetic Exercise
1. Reach under your left armpit and grasp your shoulder blade with your right hand.
2. Pull the shoulder blade forwards and up while relaxing the left shoulder complex.

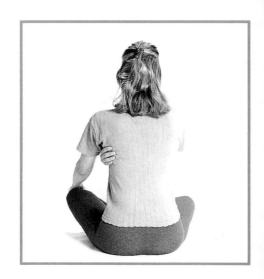

Shoulder Capsular Ligament Anterior

capsula = small box

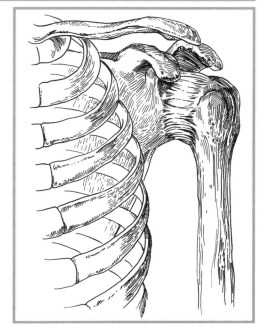

Ligament Facts
Origin:
Anterior neck of the scapula.

Insertion:
Anterior proximal head of the humerus.

Action:
Assists in the integrity of the shoulder joint.

Method of Testing
Muscle Test:
Lying on back person extends arm out to side level with shoulders, thumb towards ceiling. Press on lower forearm back and down.

Circuit Localize:
Near lung alarm point.

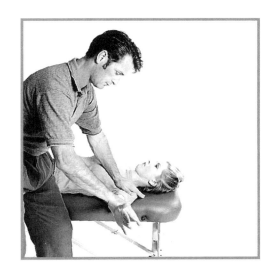

Biokinetic Exercise
1. Grasp the back of the elbow and rotate the humerus medially.
2. Firmly push the humerus into the shoulder joint and hold for at least two minutes.

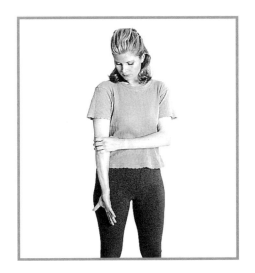

Soleus

solea = sole of foot

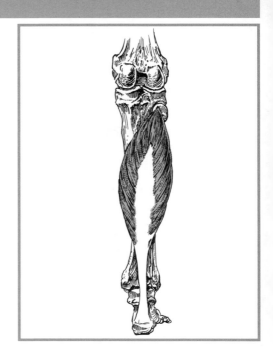

Muscle Facts

Origin:
Posterior surface of head of fibula, upper third of posterior surface of fibula, soleal line and middle third of the medial border of the tibia, and from a fibrous band between the tibia and fibula.

Insertion:
Calcaneus by way of the Achilles tendon.

Action:
Plantar flexes the foot.
Reversed Origin – Insertion Action: When standing, the calcaneus becomes the fixed origin of the muscle. The soleus muscle stabilizes the tibia on the calcaneus limiting forward sway.

Method of Testing

Muscle Test:
Client lies face down with the knee flexed to 90° and the foot in plantar flexion contracting the soleus. Pressure is against the ankle to straighten the leg while the knee is stabilized.

Or

Client lies face down with the knee bent 90°, heel flexed toward the calf of the leg. Pressure is against the heel and the sole of the foot to straighten the foot to its normal position.

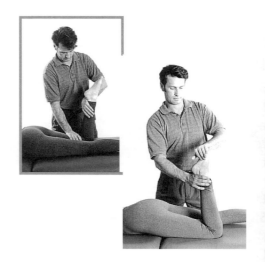

Circuit Localize:
Deeply into the middle of the posterior lower leg.

Biokinetic Exercise

1. Sit on the floor with your lower legs bent under and to the sides.
2. Grasp your heels and press very forcibly towards the inside of your knees. Rest.

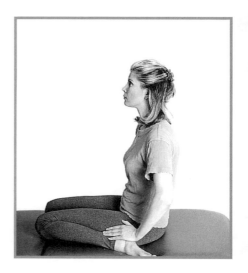

Sternocleidomastoid

sternum = breastbone; cleido = clavicle; mastoid = bone behind ear

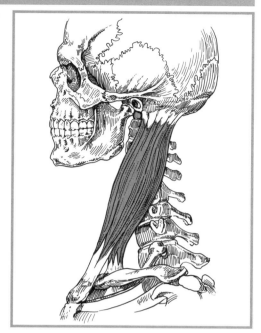

Muscle Facts
Referred to in Touch for Health as the Anterior Neck Flexors

Origin:
Sternal Head: Anterior surface of manubrium (upper bone of sternum).
Clavicular Head: Superior border and anterior surface of medial third of clavicle.

Insertion:
Lateral surface of the mastoid process of the temporal bone and lateral half of superior nuchal line of the occipital bone.

Action:
Acting unilaterally, draws the head toward the same side shoulder and rotates the head to the opposite side. Acting bilaterally, flexes the head.

Method of Testing
Muscle Test:
Lying on back client brings the chin toward the chest. Pressure is against the forehead to push it back. Other hand can protect the back of the head from injury (bilateral test). Turn the head 10° to the right and push straight back. Repeat for muscle on right.

Circuit Localize:
Sternal portion: Half way between the lower ear and the top of the sternum.
Clavicular portion: Three fingers lateral of the medial end of the clavicle and three fingers superior to the clavicle.

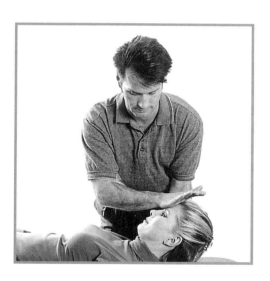

Biokinetic Exercise
1. With back straight, tilt the head forward so that the chin rests on the chest.
2. Rotate the head 10° to the right.
3. With one hand on top of your head gently press head down toward inner left collarbone.

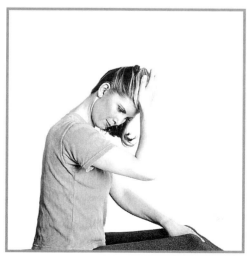

Subclavius

sub = under; clavius = clavicle

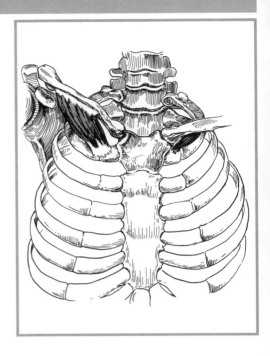

Muscle Facts

Origin:
Superior surface of the first rib, just where it joins its cartilage.

Insertion:
The groove extending along the middle half of the inferior surface of the clavicle.

Action:
Draws the clavicle downwards and forwards. Protects the sternoclavicular joint from separation in such activities as hanging by the hands.

Method of Testing

Muscle Test:
Bring the arm up alongside the ear, palm facing out. Pressure is against the forearm to bring the arm away from the head.

Circuit Localize:
Touch up and under the middle of the collar bone.

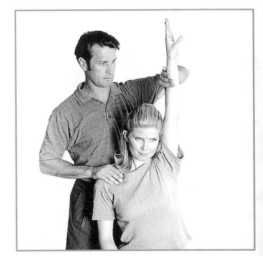

Biokinetic Exercise

1. With your right arm reaching across your front, grasp your left shoulder blade and pull in forcibly to the right, forwards and upwards.
2. Place your left hand on top of your head touching your right ear.

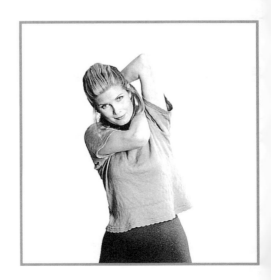

Subscapularis

sub = under; scapulae = shoulder blade

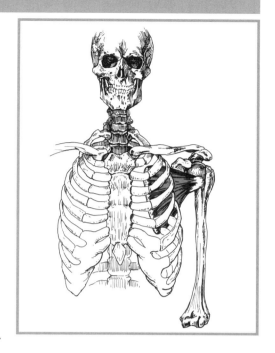

Muscle Facts
Origin:
Medial two-thirds of costal (anterior) surface of the scapula; and inferior two-thirds of groove on lateral border of the scapula.

Insertion:
The lesser tubercle of the humerus; and inferior aspect of capsule of the shoulder joint.

Action:
A prime mover for medial rotation of the humerus, being antagonistic to the infraspinatus and teres minor in this respect. Helps prevent dislocation of the shoulder joint.
Reversed Origin -- Insertion Action: When the humerus is stabilized, abducts the inferior border of the scapula.

Method of Testing
Muscle Test:
Arm out to the side, elbow flexed to 90° and level with the shoulder, hand toward the feet. Pressure is against the lower forearm to laterally rotate the humerus while stabilizing the elbow.

Circuit Localize:
Point fingertips deeply under the medial border of the scapula towards the shoulder joint.

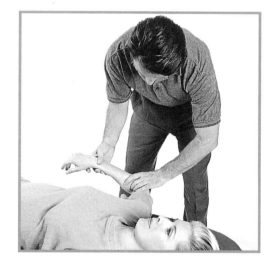

Biokinetic Exercise
1. Grasp your left shoulder blade by reaching under your left arm with your right hand.
2. Place the back of your left hand near your right shoulder blade.
3. Arch back and pull your left shoulder blade forward and up with your right hand. Rest.

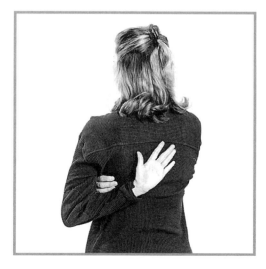

Supinator

supinator = muscle that turns palm upward or forward

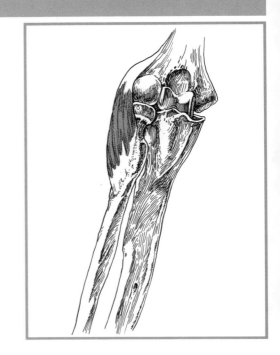

Muscle Facts

Origin:
Lateral epicondyle of humerus, ridge (supinator crest) and depression on ulna distal to radial notch, the outer parts of the ligaments of the elbow joint.

Insertion:
Lateral anterior surface of the proximal third of the radius.

Action:
Supinates the forearm, so that the palm faces forward, or anteriorly.

Method of Testing

Muscle Test:
In the Professional Kinesiology Practitioner program there are two separate tests, extemded arm or flexed arm.
Extended Arm: Hold the arm back from the side, thumb outwards. (Keep straight to immobilize biceps.) Support the humerus at the elbow to prevent shoulder rotation Pressure is at the wrist to turn the thumb inwards.
Flexed Arm: The elbow and the shoulder are both flexed so that the hand is above and behind the ear, palm toward the shoulder, thumb outwards. Support the elbow. Pressure is at the wrist to turn the thumb inwards.

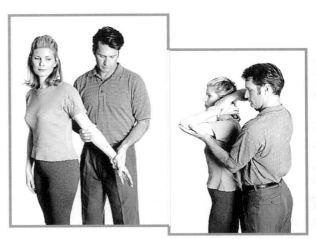

Circuit Localize:
Just below the elbow joint on the dorsal surface of the forearm.

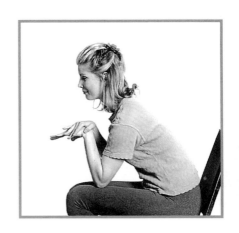

Biokinetic Exercise

1. Rest your elbow on the arm of a chair or your thigh.
2. Flex forearm 120°, fingers forward, palm down.
3. Press wrist towards elbow and rotate palm out further.

Supraspinatus

supra = above; spinatus = spine of scapula

Muscle Facts
Origin:
Medial two-thirds of fossa superior to spine of scapula.

Insertion:
Greater tubercle of humerus.

Action:
Assists deltoid muscle in abducting arm. Stabilizes the shoulder joint.

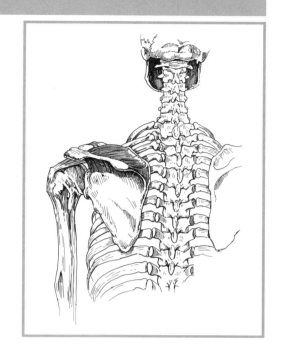

Method of Testing
Muscle Test:
Client standing or lying face up, arm is straight, about 15° forward and slightly to the side, palm facing the groin. Push toward the groin.

Circuit Localize:
Just above the spine of the scapula.

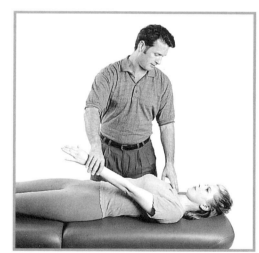

Biokinetic Exercise
1. With the back of your left hand under the chin, raise elbow up high.
2. With right hand, reach behind head and grasp left elbow.
3. Push left elbow down towards left shoulder and arch back.
4. Turn face up. Rest.

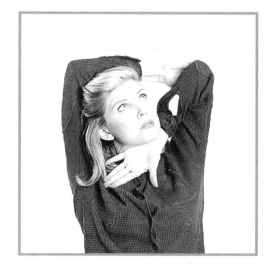

Temporalis

tempora = temples

Muscle Facts

Origin:
In a fan shape from above and behind the ear. Temporal fossa; deep surface of temporal fascia.

Insertion:
Coronoid process of mandible; anterior border of ramus of mandible nearly as far anterior as last molar tooth.

Action:
Lifts the mandible (closes mouth), clenches the teeth and retracts the lower jaw.

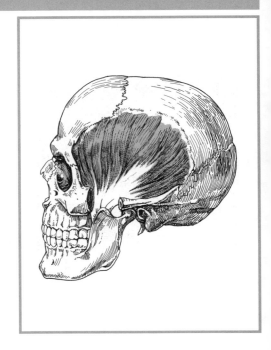

Method of Testing

Muscle Test:
Use a surrogate muscle.

Circuit Localize:
Behind, above and forward of the ear.

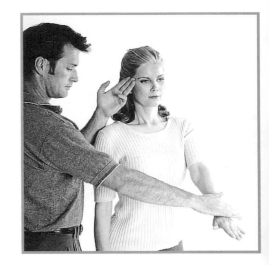

Biokinetic Exercise

There is no biokinetic exercise possible for the temporalis muscle. Instead we can balance it with flowline massage. Use your fingers to massage firmly over the entire temporalis muscle from its origin (approximately 3 fingerwidths behind to 3 fingerwidths above the ear) toward its insertion (in front of the ear) taking a number of strokes to do so.

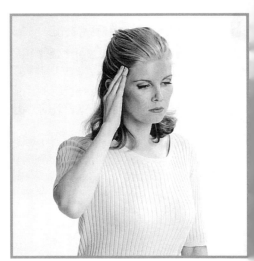

Tensor Fasciae Latae

tensor = tightener; fascia = sheath; lata = wide

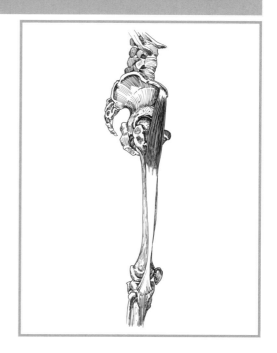

Muscle Facts
Origin:
Anterior part of outer lip of iliac crest, the lateral surface of the anterior superior iliac crest, and part of the border of the notch below it.

Insertion:
The iliotibial tract of the fascia lata of the thigh, one-fourth of the way down the outside of the thigh. The tensor fascia lata muscle lies between two layers of the fascia, and the longitudinal muscle fibers are inserted into these two layers.

Action:
A prime mover for medial rotation of the leg and an assistant for flexion and abduction of the hip joint. Stabilizes the knee laterally.

Method of Testing
Muscle Test:
Client supine. Raise leg up 45° and slightly to the side. Rotate leg medially and attempt to push it down and in towards the other leg.

Circuit Localize:
The upper lateral thigh.

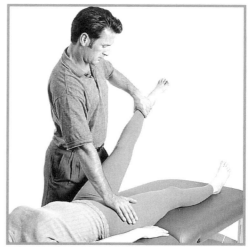

Biokinetic Exercise
1. Stand, place your left leg forward and to the side about two feet, point your feet forward.
2. Lean forwards and to the left side with your left shoulder down and your right shoulder up.
3. Place your left hand on your left hip and press it to the right and backwards. Rest.

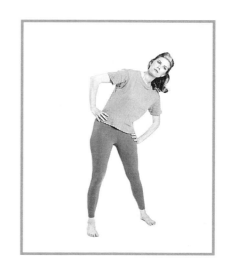

Teres Major

teres = round and smooth; major = greater

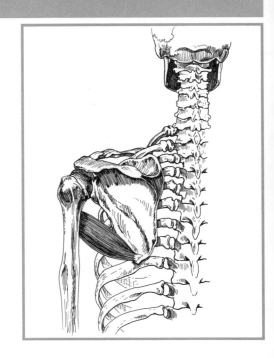

Muscle Facts
Origin:
Dorsal surface of inferior angle of scapula.

Insertion:
Crest below lesser tuberosity of humerus posterior to latissimus dorsi.

Action:
Against resistance teres major is a prime mover during inward rotation, adduction, and extension of the arm. Because its actions on the arm appear to be those of the latissimus dorsi, it has been called "the latissimus dorsi's little helper".

Method of Testing
Muscle Test:
Lying face up: With the arm bent at 90° and the fist against the lower back, draw the elbow back as far as possible. With one hand stabilizing the shoulder, push the elbow out and forward. Lying face down: With back of left hand against the lower back, and elbow up, pressure is against the elbow to push it down and out away from the back.

Circuit Localize:
Superior and lateral to the inferior angle of the scapula.

Biokinetic Exercise
1. Sitting on the floor, clasp your palms together behind you, twisting the palms backward and then down.
2. Lean back on your palms, keeping the arms straight, chest forward, and shoulders back. Rest.

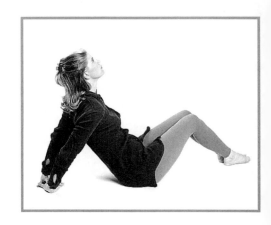

Teres Minor

teres = round and smooth; minor = lesser

Muscle Facts
Origin:
Superior two-thirds of dorsal surface of axillary border of scapula.

Insertion:
Inferior aspect of greater tubercle of the humerus and area just distal to it, posterior portion of capsule of the shoulder joint.

Action:
External rotation of humerus. Stabilization of head of humerus.
Reversed Origin – Insertion Action: When humerus is stabilized, abducts the inferior angle of the scapula.

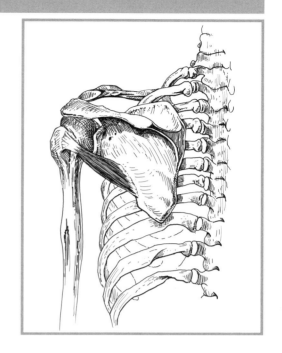

Method of Testing
Muscle Test:
The person flexes their elbow to 90° and externally rotates their humerus, keeping the elbow close to their side. Practitioner stabilizes elbow with one hand and with other pushes on wrist to internally rotate the humerus.

Circuit Localize:
Deeply on the lower lateral part of the scapula to upper end of humerus.

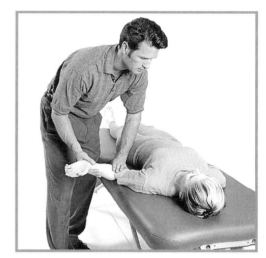

Biokinetic Exercise
1. Sitting on the floor, clasp your palms together behind you. Twist your palms up forward, and then down.
2. If you can, place your hands comfortably behind you and lean back on them, trying to keep most of your fingers interlocked.
3. Press your chest forward and shoulders back. Rest.

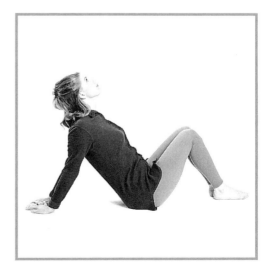

Tibialis Anterior

tibialis = pertaining to the tibia; anterior = front

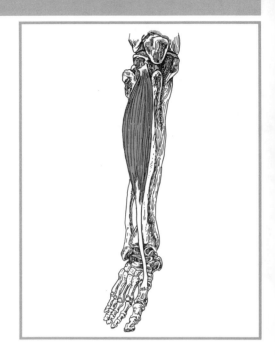

Muscle Facts

Origin:
Lateral condyle and proximal two-thirds of lateral surface of tibia and the corresponding portion of the interosseous membrane which joins the tibia and the fibula.

Insertion:
Medial and plantar surfaces of the medial cuneiform bone, plantar surface of base of first metatarsal bone.

Action:
Dorsiflexes and inverts foot at the ankle.
Reversed Origin-Insertion Action: When standing, the foot is fixed and becomes the origin. Action causes forward body lean antagonistic to the plantar flexion of the soleus and gastrocnemius. Active in the balance mechanism of anterior and posterior sway.(Bonsall, 1989)

Method of Testing

Muscle Test:
Dorsiflex the foot toward the knee and invert it (turn sole of foot inward, toward the median plane). Keep the toes curled down or straight to avoid bringing the extensor muscles of the foot into the test. Pressure is against the top inside of the foot to push it down and turn sole outward.

Circuit Localize:
Just lateral of tibia on anterior lower leg, one palm below kneecap.

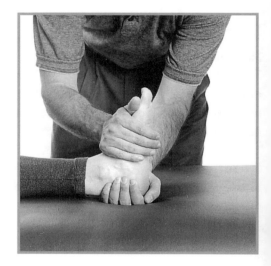

Biokinetic Exercise

1. Sit on floor with your feet in front of you and your knees up.
2. Reach around the outside of your knees and grasp the balls of your feet, turning your feet out.
3. Pull the ball and arch of your feet towards the outside of your knees.

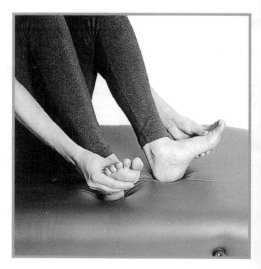

Tibialis Posterior

tibialis = pertaining to the tibia; posterior = back

Muscle Facts

Origin:
Proximal two-thirds of medial surface of fibula, lateral part of posterior surface of tibia, interosseous membrane, intermuscular septa and deep fascia.

Insertion:
Tuberosity on inferior surface of the navicular, with fibrous expansions to calcaneus, plantar surfaces of the three cuneiforms and cuboid and to bases of second, third and fourth metatarsal bones.

Action:
Prime mover for inversion; assists with plantar flexion of the foot at the ankle. Medial ankle stabilizer.

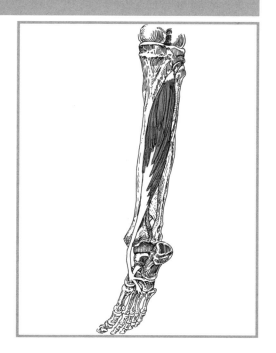

Method of Testing

Muscle Test:
Plantar flex the foot and invert the sole medially as much as possible, keeping the toes flexed. The practitioner stabilizes the leg above the ankle joint and places their other hand on the medial and lower side of the foot. Attempt to push the foot out.

Circuit Localize:
Deeply between the medial and lateral sections of the gastrocnemius in the middle third of the lower leg.

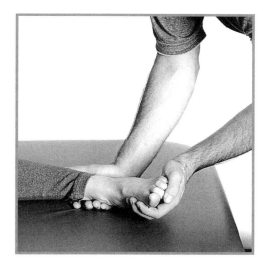

Biokinetic Exercise

1. Sit on the front edge of a chair; put your feet under you, heels up, and the toes bent under so that the tops of the toes are in contact with the floor.
2. Turn your toes in and your knees out.
3. Gently press down on your knees.

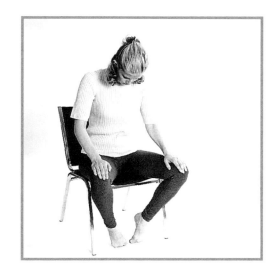

Transversus Abdominis

*transverse = muscle fibers run transversely to midline;
abdomino = belly*

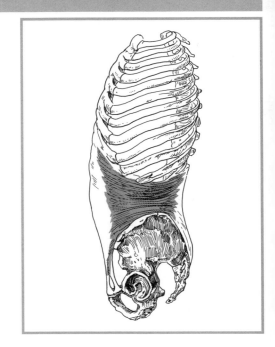

Muscle Facts

Origin:
Lateral third of the inguinal ligament, anterior three-fourths of inner lip of the iliac crest, thoracolumbar fascia, and from the inner edges of the cartilages of the last six ribs.

Insertion:
Into the linea alba by its aponeurosis which passes behind the rectus abdominis.

Action:
Constricts abdominal contents; assists in forced expiration.

Method of Testing

Muscle Test:
Observe client as he arises from a supine position. In the presence of a weak transversus abdominis, there will be bulging of the lateral abdomen (Walther, 1976).

Circuit Localize: Grasp the muscles on the side of the body midway between the bottom of the rib cage and the hips.

Biokinetic Exercise

1. Lie down on your back bending both knees together over to your left side and keeping your shoulders flat on the floor.
2. Place your knees on the floor at the imaginary points of a clock – 10:30, 9:00, 7:30. Rest at each location.

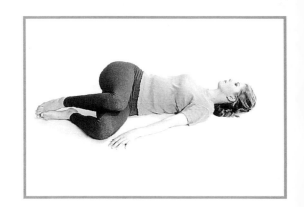

Trapezius – lower division

trapezoides = trapezoid-shaped, an irregular four sided figure

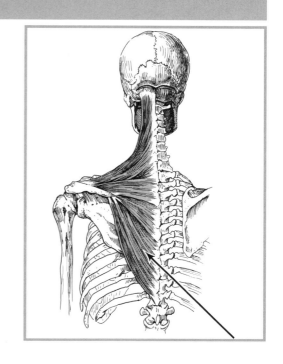

Muscle Facts
Origin:
Spinous processes of sixth – twelfth vertebrae.

Insertion:
Superior border of spine of scapula.

Action:
Depresses the scapula. Retracts the scapula. Rotates the scapula upwards so the glenoid cavity faces superiorly. Gives inferior stabilization of scapula. Aids to maintain spine in extension.

Method of Testing
Muscle Test:
Lying face up bring arm straight out to the side, palms forward. Rotate arms backwards 45 degrees. Drop arms down and back. Stabilize the shoulder. Pressure is against the back of the wrist to push the arm forward and up.

Circuit Localize:
Three thumbs lateral of T8.

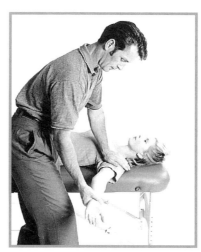

Biokinetic Exercise
Put your left palm on your sacrum and grasp your left elbow with your right hand, pulling it gently to the right. Arch back, breathe deeply, and rest.

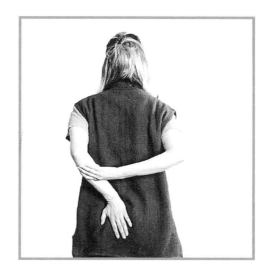

Trapezius – middle division

trapezoides = trapezoid-shaped, an irregular four sided figure

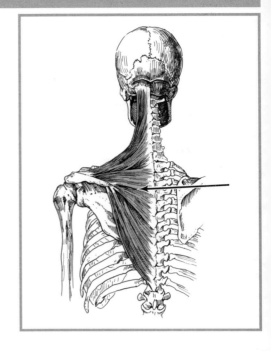

Muscle Facts
Origin:
Spinous processes of seventh cervical and upper three (or four or five) thoracic vertebrae (horizontal fibers of trapezius muscle).

Insertion:
Superior lip of posterior border of spine of scapula.

Action:
Pulls upon the spine of the scapula drawing it toward the spinal column. It is a prime mover for adduction of the scapula.

Method of Testing
Muscle Test:
Bring the arm straight out to the side and back as far as possible with the palm facing forward. Pressure is against the back of the wrist to push it forward while stabilizing the front of the shoulder.

Circuit Localize:
Three thumbs lateral of T3.

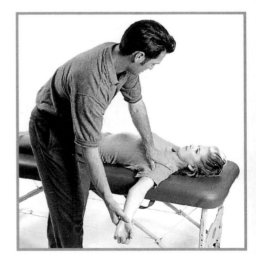

Biokinetic Exercise
Put your left palm on your bottom rib with your elbow behind you. Grasp your left elbow with your right hand, pulling it back and to the right. Arch back. Rest while breathing deeply.

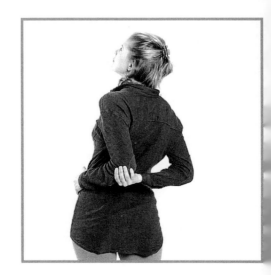

Trapezius – upper division

trapezoides = trapezoid-shaped, an irregular four sided figure

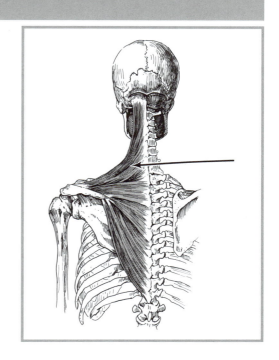

Muscle Facts
Origin:
External occipital protuberance and medial third of superior nuchal line, ligamentum nuchae and spinous process of the seventh cervical vertebra.

Insertion:
Posterior border of lateral third of clavicle and acromion process of the scapula.

Action:
Elevates the scapula as in shrugging the shoulders. Rotates the scapula upwards so the glenoid cavity faces superiorly. When acting with the other sections of the trapezius it adducts the scapula.

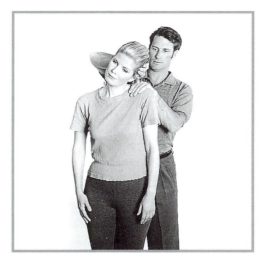

Method of Testing
Muscle Test:
Tilt the head to the side and slightly turned away from the side being tested. Bring the shoulder close to the ear leaving a little space to avoid the muscle being in a locked position. Pressure is against the shoulder and the side of the head to attempt to pull them apart.

Circuit Localize:
Midway between the head and the shoulder, pointing directly into the superficial muscle area.

Biokinetic Exercise
1. Place your left palm on your back between your shoulder blades by reaching up over your left shoulder. Keep the elbow high in the air.
2. Grasp the left elbow with your right hand by reaching behind the head.
3. Turn your face 20° to the right, and tilt your head 45° to the left. Arch back and hold.

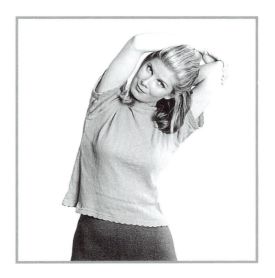

Triceps Brachii

triceps = having three heads of origin; brachii = of the arm

Muscle Facts
Origin:
Long Head: From a rough triangular depression on the scapula, immediately below the glenoid cavity (the infraglenoid tubercle).
Lateral Head: Lateral and posterior surface of humerus superior to radial groove.
Medial Head: From the distal part of the back of the humerus, over a wide space extending nearly two-thirds of the length of the bone.

Insertion:
Posterior portion of proximal surface of olecranon of the ulna and deep fascia of the forearm.

Action:
The medial head of the triceps is the prime mover for extension of the elbow joint. The long head aids in adduction and extension of the arm at the shoulder.

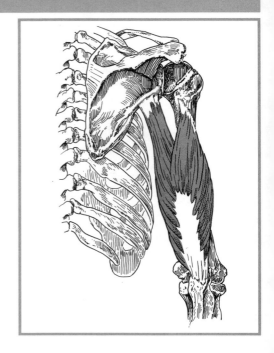

Method of Testing
Muscle Test:
Bring arm forward, palm facing front. Flex elbow about 45° so palm now faces backwards. Stabilize the elbow. Pressure is against the wrist to flex the elbow.

Circuit Localize:
Long Head: One palm below armpit on inner surface of upper arm.
Lateral Head: Along posterior distal and lateral surface of humerus.
Medial Head: On posterior distal shaft of humerus.

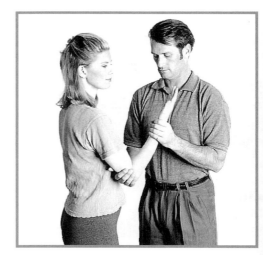

Biokinetic Exercise
Long & Lateral Heads:
1. Sit on the floor with your back near a chair.
2. Place your hands on the chair behind you with palms up and arms straight.
3. Lean and arch back.

Medial Head:
1. Sit on the floor with your legs in front of you.
2. Place your hands two feet apart behind you, about two or three feet back, depending on your size.
3. Point your fingers back and make your arms very straight (hyperextend your elbows).
4. Arch back and rest while breathing deeply.

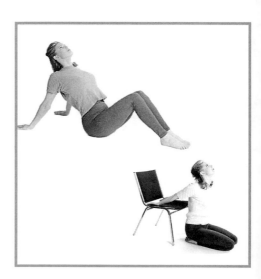

Vastus Intermedius

vastus = large; intermedius = middle

Muscle Facts

1 of the 4 muscles making up the Quadriceps.

Origin:
Anterior and lateral surfaces of proximal two-thirds of shaft of femur.

Insertion:
Forms deep part of quadriceps femoris tendon, inserting into superior border of the patella, and the patellar ligament into the tibial tuberosity.

Action:
Prime mover for knee extension.

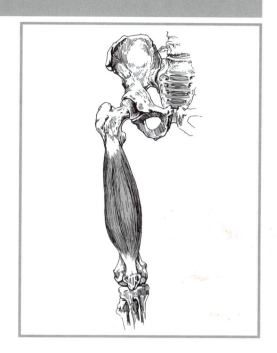

Method of Testing

Muscle Test:
Client supine, flex right knee 45° and keep right foot flat on the table. Raise left leg 50°. Practitioner places arm under the raised left leg so that his hand rests on the right knee and the left leg is supported by his arm. The foot is kept vertical and the ankle of the left leg is pressed downward.

Circuit Localize:
Deeply on the front of the thigh, midway between the hip and the knee.

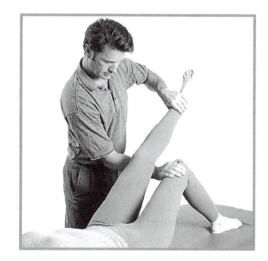

Biokinetic Exercise

1. Stand with your feet about two feet apart, pointing your feet forwards.
2. Bend forward at the hips while keeping your upper torso straight.
3. Press your knees backwards and pull up on the knee caps forcibly. Rest.

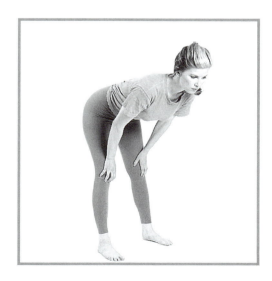

Vastus Lateralis

vastus = large; lateralis = of the side

Muscle Facts
1 of the 4 muscles making up the Quadriceps.

Origin:
Proximal portion of intertrochanteric line, anterior and inferior borders of greater trochanter, lateral lip of gluteal tuberosity, proximal half of lateral lip of linea aspera, lateral intermuscular septum, and tendon of the gluteus maximus.

Insertion:
The lateral and superior borders of the patella and the quadriceps femoris tendon.

Action:
Extends the leg at the knee and draws the patella laterally (counterbalancing the vastus medialis' diagonal pull medially, the two muscles resulting in a straight pull on the patella).

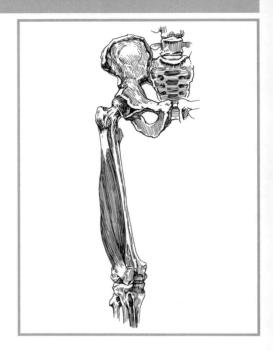

Method Of Testing
Muscle Test:
Client supine, flexes right knee 45° and keeps right foot flat on the table. Raise the left leg 50°. Practitioner places arm under the raised left leg so that his hand rests on the right knee and the left leg is supported by his arm. The foot is turned medially and the distal end of the left leg is pressed downward, and slightly medial.

Circuit Localize:
Lateral aspect of anterior thigh halfway between hip and knee.

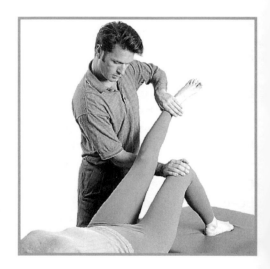

Biokinetic Exercise
Stand with your legs about two feet apart and turn your left foot in 45°. Hyperextend your knee, bend forward and slightly to the left and pull up forcibly on the knee cap.

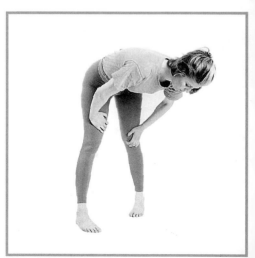

Vastus Medialis

vastus = large; medialis = of the middle

Muscle Facts
1 of the 4 muscles making up the Quadriceps.

Origin:
Distal half of intertrochanteric line, medial lip of linea aspera and proximal part of medial supracondylar ridge, medial intermuscular septum, tendons of adductor magnus and adductor longus.

Insertion:
Medial border of the patella and the quadriceps femoris tendon into the tibial tuberosity.

Action:
Extends the leg at the knee and draws the patella medially (counterbalancing the vastus lateralis' diagonal pull laterally, the two muscles resulting in a straight pull on the patella).

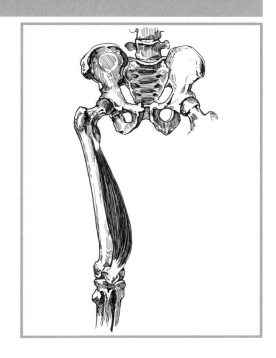

Method of Testing
Muscle Test:
Client supine, flex right knee 45° and keep right foot flat on the table. Raise left leg 50°. Practitioner places arm under the raised left leg so that his hand rests on the right knee and the left leg is supported by his arm. The foot is turned laterally and the ankle of the left leg is pressed downward and slightly lateral.

Circuit Localize:
One palm width superior of the knee on the medial side of the thigh.

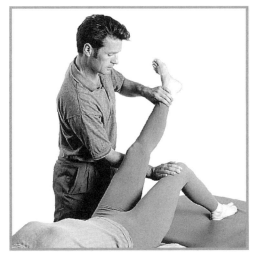

Biokinetic Exercise
1. Stand with your feet about two feet apart, turn your feet out about 80°.
2. Bend forward at the hips while keeping your upper torso straight and pull up on your knee caps. Rest.

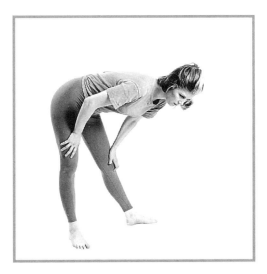

Part III

Appendix A
Appendix B
References
Index

Appendix A: Glossary Of Terms

Directional Terms

ANTERIOR: Nearer to the front; at the front of the
(Ventral) body.

CENTRAL: Nearer to or toward the center.

DEEP: Away from the surface of the body;
(Internal) inner.

DISTAL: Farthest from the center, from the
medial line, or from the trunk.

INFERIOR: Away from the head; nearer to the
(Caudal) feet; lower part of a structure;
generally refers to structures
in the trunk.

LATERAL: Farther from the midline of the body
or a structure; at or belonging to the
side.

MEDIAL: Nearer the midline of the body or a
structure.

PERIPHERAL:
Farther from or away from the center.

POSTERIOR: Nearer to the back; at the back of the
(Dorsal) body; top surface of the foot.

PROXIMAL: The end nearest to the center of the
body, or the trunk.

SUPERFICIAL:
Toward or on the surface of the body;
(External) outer.

SUPERIOR: Toward the head: the upper of two
(Cranial) parts; generally refers to structures
in the trunk.

Terms Of Movement

ABDUCTION: Movement away from the median
plane or axis of the trunk, as in
raising arms to the side horizontally
and scapula away from the spinal
column.

ADDUCTION: Movement toward the median plane
or axis of the trunk, as in lowering
arms to the side.

DEPRESSION: Moving a body part inferiorly, e.g.,
lowering the shoulder.

DORSIFLEXION: Flexes top of foot upwards.

ELEVATION: Moving a body part superiorly, e.g.,
raising the shoulder.

EVERSION: Turning sole of foot outwards;
weight on inner edge of foot.

EXTENSION: Straightening or increasing the
angle between body parts, as in
elbow joint when hand moves away
from shoulder. In the shoulder and
hip joints, a return movement of
the humerus or femur downward.

FLEXION: Bending or decreasing the angle
between body parts, e.g., flexing
the elbow joint by bringing the
hand to the shoulder. At the shoulder and hip joints, movement of the
humerus or femur to the front and
upward is considered flexion.

INVERSION: Turning sole of foot inward, toward
the median plane; weight on outer
edge of foot.

PLANTAR FLEXION:
Movement of sole of foot downward.

Appendix A: Glossary Of Terms

PRONATION: Rotating the forearm medially so that palm faces downward or posteriorly.

PROTRACTION: Movement along a plane parallel to the ground and away from the midline.

RETRACTION: Movement along a plane parallel to the ground and toward the midline.

ROTATION: Moving around the long axis. **Internal rotation** or **medial rotation:** Rotation toward body, as when humerus is turned inward. **External rotation** or **lateral rotation:** Rotation away from the body, as when humerus is turned outward.

SUPINATION: Rotating the forearm laterally so that palm turns upwards or anteriorly.

Miscellaneous Anatomical Terms

ACETABULUM: The rounded cavity of the external surface of the innominate bone that receives the head of the femur.

AGONIST: Muscle that shortens to perform a movement.

ANTAGONIST: A muscle that relaxes to allow the agonist to perform a movement.

APONEUROSIS: A broad glistening sheet of tendon-like tissue which serves to invest and attach muscles to each other, and also to the parts which they move.

AXILLA: The armpit.

CARPUS: The wrist consisting of eight small bones arranged in two rows – carpal, adj.

CONDYLE: A large, rounded eminence at the articular end of a bone.

COSTA: Rib

CREST: A prominent border or ridge on a bone.

EPICONDYLE:

A prominence above a condyle.

FASCIA: Sheath

FOSSA: A depression in or on a bone.

GROOVE: A furrow in the bone that accommodates a soft structure such as a blood vessel, nerve, or tendon.

HYPER: Too much

Appendix A: Glossary Of Terms

HYPO: Too little

INSERTION: The end of a muscle attached to the bone and/or tissue it moves.

INTER: Between

INTRA: Inside

LINE: A less prominent ridge than a crest.

MAJOR: Bigger, greater

MALLEOLUS: A part or process of a bone shaped like a hammer. External malleolus, at the lower end of the fibula. Internal malleolus, situated at the lower end of the tibia.

METACARPUS: The five bones which form that part of the hand between the wrist and fingers – metacarpal, adj.

METATARSUS: The five bones of the foot between the ankle and the toes – metatarsal, adj.

MINOR: Smaller, lesser

ORIGIN: The end of a muscle that remains relatively fixed during contraction of that muscle.

PHALANGES: The individual finger and toe bones, two or three per digit – Phalanx, singular; phalangeal, adj.

PLANTAR: Pertaining to the sole of the foot, e.g. plantar flexion, downward movement of the great toe.

PROCESS: A prominent, roughened projection, e.g., spinous process of a vertebra.

PRONE: Lying face-down, or forearm and hand with the palm side downward.

PROPRIOCEPTOR: One of a variety of sensory end organs (such as the muscle spindle and the Golgi's tendon organ) in muscles, tendons, and joint capsules.

SUBLUXATION: Incomplete dislocation of a joint, e.g. vertebrae out of alignment.

SUPINE: Lying on the back, or forearm and hand turned with the palm upward.

SUPRA: Above, over

TARSUS: The seven small bones of the foot tarsal, adj.

TROCHANTER: A large, blunt projection found only on the femur.

TUBERCLE: A small, rounded process.

TUBEROSITY: A large, rounded, usually roughened process.

Appendix B: Muscle Monintoring Review

Review of Procedures

Muscle testing or muscle monitoring makes the use of biokinetic exercises more exact in three major ways:

1. It allows us to identify what type of tissue is out of balance – muscle, tendon, ligament or fascia. This then lets us know how long we should hold the biokinetic exercise position.

2. It allows us to identify how the tissue is out of balance – weak or hypotonic; too tight or hypertonic. After the exercise, muscle monitoring can confirm that the tissues are now in balance.

3. It allows us to find the optimum position for the biokinetic exercise.

First we shall describe two indicator muscles and the corrections required should one or both be out of balance. Then we shall go through some basic clearing tests to ensure that we are getting accurate feedback from the indicator muscles.

What Is Muscle Monitoring?

While the biokinetic exercises can be done without needing to use muscle monitoring, knowing how to use muscle monitoring can give us valuable information about the type of tissue and how it is out of balance so it is a wonderful biofeedback tool.

In muscle monitoring we place a specific muscle in its contracted position isolating it as much as possible from its neighboring muscles. We then attempt to extend the muscle to see whether it locks or unlocks. We are not testing the strength of the muscle, but rather the integrity or quality of the muscle-to-brain and brain-to-muscle circuitry. For this type of muscle monitoring we don't need a lot of pressure. One of the keys is to increase the pressure gradually from minimum to a maximum of 2–5 pounds over a period of about two seconds looking to see if the muscle locks or gives way.

Muscles can be out of balance for a number of different reasons including, but not limited to, nutrient deficiencies, emotional stress, toxicity, injury, dehydration, sensitivities to colors, metals, etc. For this reason we'll describe two simple muscles which can be used. Because they are used as biofeedback to indicate something about how the body is functioning, we refer to them as **indicator muscles** (IM). If one isn't suitable for muscle monitoring, you can use the other. Sometimes they may be unlocked when monitored "in the clear" so we describe some corrections from Touch for Health that you can use to balance them.

A. **DELTOID** (actually Middle Deltoid; see page 33)

This muscle is delta-shaped, caps the shoulder, and is responsible for moving the arm laterally away from the side of the body. The client or testee extends their arm horizontally to the side of the body, palm down. The facilitator or testor places his hand over client's wrist, or lower forearm just above the wrist, and gently attempts to push the arm down toward the side while the other hand rests comfortably on client's other shoulder.

Until you become really comfortable with muscle monitoring you may want to follow the procedure outlined below:

1. Ask the person being muscle monitored (testee) if there is any reason why you cannot work with them. Maybe they have a recent injury that would make muscle monitoring inadvisable.

2. Inform the testee that he/she should let you know immediately if they feel any pain during the monitoring and to let the arm go to prevent any injury.

3. Place your other hand on the testee's other shoulder to increase the stability for both of you.

Appendix B: Muscle Monintoring Review

4. Demonstrate the range of motion of the muscle you are about to monitor. This lets the testee's brain know which particular energy circuit is about to be monitored.

5. Let the testee know that you'll tell them to "Hold", then you'll attempt to push the arm down.

6. Say "Hold". With your monitoring hand already on the testee's wrist or lower forearm, increase your pressure from zero to a maximum of 2–5 pounds then release, all in the space of about two seconds. You are interested only in what happens in the first one to two inches. If the muscle circuit is "switched on" or has integrity it will lock in position. If it is "switched off", it may unlock, appear to be mushy or "bounce".

B. **ANTERIOR DELTOID** (see page 32)

This is the anterior portion of the delta-shaped deltoid muscle. With the arm down by the side, contraction of this muscle would raise the arm forwards. To monitor the anterior deltoid we place the straight arm directly over the thigh at a 45° angle, palm down, and apply pressure over the wrist or lower forearm attempting to push it toward the thigh. Apart from the different starting position and monitoring direction all other muscle monitoring procedures are the same as outlined previously for the deltoid muscle.

Techniques to Balance the Deltoid Muscle

Sometimes the indicator muscle we want to use may be switched off in the clear. Below we have described some simple procedures from Touch for Health to balance the muscle so it can be used as an I.M.

1. **Spinal Vertebrae Reflex Technique:** (for bilateral weakness of deltoid muscles) Massage

skin rapidly, but gently, for 10–30 seconds back and forth in a head-to-foot motion over the spinal processes of vertebrae T3 and T4.

For unilateral or bilateral weaknesses of the deltoid muscles one or both of the corrections below can be used:

2. **Front Neuro-Lymphatic Points:** Between 3–4 and 4–5 ribs near the breastbone. Deep massage for 20–30 seconds.

   Back Neuro-Lymphatic Points: Between T3–4 and T4–5, one inch to each side of the spine. Deep massage for 20–30 seconds.

3. **Neuro-Vascular Holding Points:** Anterior fontanel, the baby's soft spot on the top of the head. Hold lightly for 20–30 seconds.

Techniques to Balance the Anterior Deltoid Muscle

1. **Spinal Vertebrae Reflex Technique:** (for bilateral weakness of anterior deltoid muscles) Massage skin rapidly, but gently, for 10–30 seconds back and forth in a head-to-foot motion over the spinal process of vertebrae T4.

For unilateral or bilateral weaknesses of the anterior deltoid muscles one or both of the corrections below can be used:

2. **Front Neuro-Lymphatic Points:** Between 3–4 and 4–5 ribs near the breastbone. Deep massage for 20–30 seconds.

   Back Neuro-Lymphatic Points: Between T3–4 and T4–5, one inch to each side of the spine. Deep massage for 20–30 seconds.

3. **Neuro-Vascular Holding Points:** Anterior fontanel, the baby's soft spot on the top of the head. Hold lightly for 20–30 seconds.

Appendix B: Muscle Monintoring Review

Testing for a "Balanced Indicator Muscle"

PRINCIPLE
Certain tests are required to ensure that the indicator muscles you will be using are in proprioceptive homeostasis. Otherwise manual muscle monitoring or circuit localizing could give you inaccurate feedback.

METHOD
The same muscle on both sides of the body, when monitored, must individually or simultaneously demonstrate proprioceptive homeostasis as defined by points 1 through 4 below.

1.   The muscles must lock when monitored in contraction.

2.   The muscles must lock when tested in extension (monitoring their antagonists as a group).

If the muscles unlock in steps 1 or 2, use neuro-lymphatic reflexes and neuro-vascular holding points to balance the muscles.

3.   (a)   Now **sedate** the muscle spindle cells for the same muscle on both sides of the body by pushing the fingers together in the belly of the muscles. Both muscles should now unlock when monitored in contraction, and when placed in extension the antagonist muscles should also unlock.

      (b)   Now **tonify** the spindle cells by pulling apart in the middle of the contracted muscles. The muscles should now lock in contraction, and in extension their antagonists should also lock.

4.   Instead of step 3, a magnet can be used to test that the indicator muscles are in proprioceptive

homeostasis.

(a)   The muscle must unlock when the north pole of a magnet is applied to the belly of the muscle when monitored in contraction.

(b)   The muscle must unlock when the south pole of a magnet is applied to the belly of the muscle when monitored in extension.

If the muscles don't respond as described in steps 3 and/or 4, the person may be 'uptight' or in 'mental override'. Have the person breathe deeply, drop and relax their shoulders, then repeat steps 3 and/or 4.

Pre-checks and Corrections for Accurate Indicator Muscle Biofeedback

I.   Hydration: the Hair Tug Test

Test: Client or practitioner gently pulls a tuft of hair (to stretch the skin) while the practitioner monitors a balanced indicator muscle.

Correction: If indicator muscle unlocks, client drinks some water. Practitioner checks to see that I.M. now remains locked when the hair is tugged.

II.   Switching

Test:
1.   Practitioner monitors any switched-on muscle using one hand.

2.   He/she immediately monitors the same muscle using the other hand.

3.   Practitioner immediately retests muscle with the first hand.

If the muscle unlocks on the second or third test, we

130

Appendix B: Muscle Monintoring Review

assume a switched condition.

4. Practitioner monitors one I.M. with one hand and the same I.M. on the other side of the body with their other hand simultaneously.

5. Practitioner changes hands to remonitor both I.M.s.

6. Practitioner uncrosses hands to remonitor both muscles as in step 4.

If the muscles unlock on the second or third tests (steps 5 or 6), we assume a switched condition.

Correction:

1. Client places one hand over the navel.

2. With the other hand, firmly massage two points, one on either side of the top of the breast bone (sternum), and below and slightly to the outside of the inner ends of the collar bones, (K27 acupuncture points), for 20–30 seconds.

3. Change hands and repeat steps 1 and 2, if you wish.

4. With one hand over navel, client massages below lower lip (CV24, the approximate end of the central meridian) and above the upper lip (GV 26, the approximate end of the governing meridian) with the other hand for 20–30 seconds.

5. Change hands and repeat step 4, if you wish.

6. With one hand over navel, client massages GV1 (at the base of the tailbone) for 20–30 seconds.

7. Change hands and repeat step 6, if you

wish.

8. Repeat **Switching Tests** (steps 1–6) to ensure that corrections have been accomplished.

III. SWITCHING: A VERBAL TEST

1. Client says 'yes' then practitioner monitors a balanced indicator muscle. Should remain locked.

2. Client says 'no'. The indicator muscle should now unlock.

3. (a) Locked on 'yes', unlocked on 'no' = no switching is present.

   (b) Unlocked on 'yes', locked on 'no' = switching is present. Correct as described earlier in 2.

   (c) If indicator muscles are locked on both 'yes' and 'no', or unlocked on both 'yes' and 'no', client can do emotional stress release regarding muscle monitoring, being touched, being willing to be vulnerable, staying present, resisting less, etc.

IV. ELECTROMAGNETIC SCREENING TEST

Test a balanced indicator muscle while touching the client's torso with the tips of all five fingers. If I.M. unlocks, one or more electromagnetic imbalances are present.

Correction: Five Finger Quick Fix

1. Place all five fingertips of one hand around client's navel with thumb uppermost and keep them there while doing steps 2, 3,

Appendix B: Muscle Monintoring Review

and 4 with the other hand.

2. Massage in the two hollows immediately below and slightly lateral to the inner ends of the collarbones (K27s, Brain Buttons).

3. Massage on the midline, just below the lower lip.

4. Massage on the midline, just above the upper lip.

V.   OVER ENERGY

Method:
1. Test a balanced indicator muscle in the clear.

2. Practitioner runs his/her hand smoothly up the front of the body from the pubic bone to the lower lip ('zip-up').

3. Retest the muscle.

4. Run your hand down the front of the body from the lower lip to the pubic bone ('zip-down').

5. Retest the muscle.

6. If the muscle remains switched on when you run up the meridian and is switched off when you run down, the central meridian is responding as it should.

7. If the muscle switches off when you run your hand up the meridian and/or remains switched on when you run your hand down the meridian, proceed to the correction below.

Correction: CV7

1. Brush up over an acupressure point (CV7), one inch below navel.

2. Repeat steps 1–5 of the method. If the central meridian is now working correctly, massage CV7 for about 20 seconds for a longer-lasting correction.

Correction: Cook's Hookups
This technique, named after its developer, the late Wayne Cook, is in two parts:

Part A

1. While sitting, place your left foot on your right knee.

2. Place your right hand on your left ankle.

3. Place palm of left hand under ball of left foot.

4. Place tongue against roof of mouth just behind the front teeth. With lips closed, breathe in through nose.

5. On the out-breath, open mouth and let tongue fall behind the bottom front teeth.

6. Continue this breathing pattern for at least one minute.

Part B

1. Seated with both feet flat on the floor, place tips of fingers and thumbs together.

2. Continue breathing as in the first position.

3. Maintain this position for at least one

Appendix B: Muscle Monintoring Review

minute.

Part C

1. Repeat the earlier muscle tests.

2. Zip up meridian:
   Correct response = locked
   Incorrect response = unlocked

3. Zip down meridian:
   Correct response = unlocked
   Incorrect response = locked

VI. AURICULARS

Test:
1. Practitioner monitors client's I.M.

2. Client turns head to left and I.M. is monitored.

3. Client turns head to right side and I.M. is monitored again.

Correction:
1. If I.M. unlocks when head is turned to one side client or practitioner unfolds that ear three times.

2. Repeat pretests to see if correction has been effective.

VII. EYE DIRECTIONS

Test:
1. Practitioner monitors client's I.M.

2. Client keeps head directed forwards and looks to the left with the eyes while I.M. is monitored.

3. Client looks to the right with the eyes while I.M. is monitored.

Correction:
If the I.M. switched off in steps 2 or 3 above, client places one hand over navel and massages K27s with the other hand. For a more powerful correction client can track their eyes repeatedly from left to right while doing the correction.

References

Barton, John. "Biokinetic Exercises for the Low Back". *Creative Health* 5, (6) October-November 1991.

Biokinesiology Institute. *Be Your Own Chiropractor Through Biokinetic Exercises.* 2nd ed. Biokinesiology Institute, U.S.A.: 1979.

Biokinesiology Institute. *The Atlas.* East Longmeadow, Massachusetts: Celecom, 1981.

Bonsall, Andrew Paul. *Flash Anatomy Cards: The Muscles.* 2nd ed. U.S.A.: Flash Anatomy Inc., 1989.

Daniels, Lucille and Catherine Worthingham. *Muscle Testing: Techniques of Manual Examination.* Philadelphia, Pennsylvania: W.B. Saunders Co., 1980.

Dewe, Bruce A.J. and Joan Dewe. *Professional Health Provider I: Advanced Specialized Kinesiology Methods.* Auckland, New Zealand: Professional Health Practice Workshops, May 1990.

Gray, Henry. *Gray's Anatomy.* A revised American edition, from the 15th English edition. New York: Bounty Books, 1977.

Lippert, Lynn. *Clinical Kinesiology for Physical Therapy Assistants.* 2nd ed. Philadelphia, Pennsylvania: F.A. Davis Co., 1994.

Rasch, Philip J. and Roger K. Burke. *Kinesiology and Applied Anatomy.* 6th ed. Philadelphia, Pennsylvania: Lea & Febiger, 1978.

Thie, John F. *Touch for Health.* rev. ed. Sherman Oaks, California: T.H. Enterprises, 1994.

Topping, Wayne W. *Biokinesiology Workbook.* Bellingham, Washington: Topping International Institute, 1985.

Tortora, Gerard J. and Nicholas P. Anagnostakos. *Principles of Anatomy & Physiology.* 2nd ed. New York: Harper & Row, 1978.

Walther, David S. *Applied Kinesiology, The Advanced Approach to Chiropractic.* Pueblo, Colorado: Systems DC, 1976.

Index

A

abdominal oblique external, 44
abdominal oblique internal, 62
abdominal transversalis, 116
abdominals, 19
abduction, 125
abductor hallucis, 22
acetabulum, 126
adduction, 124
adductor brevis, 23
adductor longus, 24
adductor magnus, 25
adductor pollicis, 26
agonist, 126
antagonist, 126
antagonist tissues, 17, 130
anterior, 125
anterior deltoid,   19, 32, 129
anterior neck flexors, 14, 15
aponeurosis, 126
Atlas, 9
auriculars, 133
axilla, 125

B

Barton, John and Margaret, 9
Be Your Own Chiropractor, 9
biceps brachii, 27
biceps femoris, 28
Biokinesiology, 9, 17, 19, 63, 88, 102
Biokinesiology Institute, 9
biokinetic exercises, 9, 19, 20, 128
blood sugar imbalances, 63
brachioradialis, 28
buccinator, 30

C

carpus, 126
caudal, 125

central, 125
central meridian, 16, 17, 131, 132
circuit localizing, 9, 16, 17, 19, 20
condyle, 126
contracted position of a muscle, 19, 130
Cook, Wayne, 132
Cooks Hookups, 132
coracobrachialis, 31
costa, 126
cranial, 125
crest, 126
CV 7, 132
CV 24, 131

D

deep, 125
deltoid, 31, 128
deltoid anterior, 19, 32, 128, 129
deltoid middle, 19, 33, 128, 129
deltoid posterior, 19, 34
depression, 108, 125
diaphragm, 35, 108
directional terms, 125
distal, 125
dorsal, 125
dorsal interossei, 36
dorsiflexion, 125

E

Edu-Kinesthetics, 20
electromagnetic screening test, 131
elevation, 125
emotional stress release, 10
epicondyle, 126
eversion, 125
extension, 125, 130
extensor carpi radialis longus, 37
extensor carpi ulnaris, 38
extensor digitorum brevis, 39, 41
extensor digitorum longus, 40

135

Index

extensor hallucis brevis, 39, 41
extensor hallucis longus, 42
extensor pollicis longus, 43
external, 125
external abdominal oblique, 20, 44
external oblique, 20, 44
external oblique abdominal, 20, 44
external pterygoid, 84
eye directions, 133

F

fascia, 9, 10, 16, 20, 126
fascia lata, 111
fetal position, 9
five finger quick fix, 131, 132
flexion, 125
flexor carpi radialis, 37, 45
flexor carpi ulnaris, 46
flexor digitorum brevis, 47
flexor digitorum longus, 48
flexor digitorum profundus, 49, 50
flexor digitorum sublimis, 50
flexor digitorum superficialis, 50
flexor hallucis brevis, 51
flexor hallucis longus, 52
flexor pollicis brevis, 53
flexor pollicis longus, 54
flowline massage, 110
fossa, 126

G

gastrocnemius, 55
gluteus maximus, 56, 88
gluteus medius, 57
gluteus minimus, 58
Goodheart, George, 10
gracilis, 59
groove, 107, 126
GV 1, 131
GV 26, 131

H

hair tug test, 130
hamstrings, 28, 88, 99, 100
headaches, 15
hydration test, 130
hyper, 126
hypertonic muscles, 9, 10
hypo, 127
hypotonic muscles, 9, 10

I

iliacus, 60, 83
indicator muscle, 17, 129, 130
inferior, 125
infraspinatus, 61, 107
insertion, 9, 19, 127
inter, 127
internal, 125
internal abdominal oblique, 62
internal oblique, 62
internal pterygoid, 85
interossei dorsales, 36
interossei plantares, 79
intra, 127
inversion, 125

J, K

kinetic tissues, 9
K27, 131, 133

L

lateral, 125
latissimus dorsi, 63, 112
latissimus dorsi tendon, 63
levator scapulae, 14, 15, 64
ligament, 9, 10, 16, 17
line, 127

Index

low back, 9, 10, 12, 19
lumbricals (of foot), 65
lumbricals (of hand), 66

M

magnet, 130
major, 127
malleolus, 127
masseter, 67
medial, 125
metacarpus, 127
metatarsus, 127
middle deltoid, 19, 33
minor, 127
multifidus spinea superficial, 12, 13
muscle, 9, 10, 17, 19
  deep, 16
  surface, 16
muscle monitoring, 128, 129
muscle testing, 20

N

neck, 14, 15, 19
neuro-lymphatic points, 129
neuro-vascular holding points, 129

O

obliquus abdominis internus, 62
obliquus capitis inferior, 68
obliquus capitis superior, 69
obliquus externus abdominis, 19, 44
obliquus internus abdominis, 62
opponens digiti minimi, 70
opponens minimi digiti, 70
opponens pollicis, 71
optimum position for biokinetic exercise, 17, 20
origin, 9, 19, 127
over energy, 132

"overstressed" tissue, 16, 17, 19

P

pain, 9, 10, 11
palm, 10
palmaris longus, 72
pectineus, 73
pectoralis major clavicular, 74, 75
pectoralis major sternal, 75
pectoralis minor, 76
peripheral, 125
peroneus tertius, 77
phalanges, 127
piriformis, 78
plantar, 127
plantar flexion, 125
plantar interossei, 79
popliteus, 80
posterior, 125
process, 127
Professional Kinesiology Practitioner I, 9, 19, 20, 108
pronation, 126
pronator quadratus, 81
pronator teres, 82
prone, 127
proprioceptive homeostasis, 130
proprioceptor, 10, 127
protraction, 126
proximal, 125
psoas major, 9, 10, 83
pterygoid lateral, 84
pterygoid medial, 85
pyramidalis, 86

Q

quadratus lumborum, 12, 13, 87
quadriceps, 93, 121, 122, 123

137

Index

R

rectus abdominis, 88
rectus capitis anterior, 89
rectus capitis lateralis, 20, 90
rectus capitis posterior, 20
rectus capitis posterior major, 91
rectus capitis posterior minor, 91, 92
rectus femoris, 93
reflex action, 10
retraction, 126
rhomboid major, 18, 94, 101
rhomboid minor, 95
rotation, 126
rotatores brevis, 96
rotatores longus, 97

S

sartorius, 98
seesaw analogy, 17
semimembranosus, 99
semitendinosus, 100
serratus anterior, 101
serratus anterior #5 (tendon), 102
serratus posterior inferior, 12, 13
shoulder capsular ligament anterior, 103
shoulders, 14, 15, 19
soleus, 104
spinal vertebrae reflex technique, 129
spindle cells, 10, 16, 130
sternocleidomastoid, 14, 15, 105
subclavius, 106
subluxation, 127
subscapularis, 107
superficial, 125
superior, 125
supination, 126
supinator, 108
supine, 127
supra, 127
supraspinatus, 109
surrogate muscle, 20
switching, 131, 132

T

tarsus, 127
temporalis, 110
tendon, 9, 10, 16, 17, 18
tensor fasciae latae, 111
teres major, 112
teres minor, 107, 113
therapy localizing, 19
tibialis anterior, 114
tibialis posterior, 115
times to hold biokinetic positions, 10
Touch for Health, 9, 19, 20, 105, 129
transversus abdominis, 116
trapezius, lower division, 117
trapezius, middle division, 101,118
trapezius, upper division, 14, 15, 119
triceps brachii, 120
trochanter, 127
tubercle, 127
tuberosity, 127

U

upper trapezius, 14, 15

V

vastus intermedius, 121
vastus lateralis, 122, 123
vastus medialis, 122, 123
ventral, 125

W

"weak" tissues, 16, 17, 19

X, Y, Z

Books for Balancing Your Life Naturally

Allergies–How to Find and Conquer
by Biokinesiology Institute

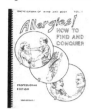

Teaches muscle testing to identify vitamins, minerals foods, non-food items such as feathers, light, plastic, wood, and wool to which a person is sensitive. How to correct such allergies through use of emotions and nutrition. Wire spiral bound. 143 pp. $20.00

Balancing the Body's Energies
by Dr. Wayne W Topping

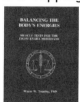

The eight extra meridians of Chinese acupuncture relate to organs including hypothalamus, pineal, thymus, anterior and posterior pituitary, and regulate the 12 regular meridians. This book describes 35 muscle tests, including eight indicator muscles that can balance all 20 meridians. 121 pp. $16.00

Biokinesiology Workbook
by Dr. Wayne W. Topping

This manual provides a useful and extensive summary of many of the basic techniques of Biokinesiology. Learn how to therapy localize imbalanced tissues and organ reflexes, how to determine which nutrition will correct these imbalances, food and environmental sensitivity testing, how to use flowline massage and acupressure points and emotional balancing. Spiral bound. 111 pp. $21.00

Stress Release
by Dr. Wayne W. Topping

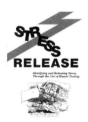

Muscle testing is a simple yet very effective, biofeedback tool to identify what is creating stress for the individual. Learn how to defuse emotional distress, to test for and correct lack of agreement between left and right brain hemispheres, and to apply these and other techniques to creating change – in weight, self-esteem, severe illness, and entrenched habits. Learn which emotions are associated with which organ functions and how to correct emotional imbalances.
163 pp. $13.00

Success Over Distress
by Dr. Wayne W. Topping

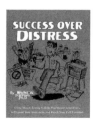

Reducing stress today prevents tomorrow's illnesses! Effective stress management requires: 1) knowledge of what stress is and ways to identify stressors; 2) knowledge of how to eliminate, reduce or modify stressors; 3) a willingness to make appropriate changes. Only you can decide to change. This book makes it easier, however, by describing stress and by providing many stress management techniques that are made more effective through the use of muscle testing biofeedback. 163 pp. $16.00

Product Order Form

	Allergies - How to Find and Conquer – Biokinesiology Institute	$ 20.00	
	Balancing the Body's Energies – Wayne W. Topping	$ 16.00	
	Biokinesiology Workbook – Wayne W. Topping	$ 21.00	
	Stress Release – Wayne W. Topping	$ 13.00	
	Success Over Distress – Wayne W. Topping	$ 16.00	
	Other Good Resources		
	Brain Gym – Paul & Gail Dennison	$ 9.00	
	Brain Gym Teacher's Edition – Paul & Gail Dennison	$ 20.00	
	Let's Play Doctor! – Joel D. Wallach & Ma Lan	$ 12.95	
	Making the Brain/Body Connection – Sharon Promislow	$ 18.95	
	Rare Earths – Joel D. Wallach & Ma Lan	$ 19.95	
	Your Body's Many Cries for Water – Feyedoon Batmanghelidj	$ 14.95	

* Shipping costs: Add $4.00 per item book rate
   or $4.50 per item priority mail
 For Foreign orders: Add $7.00 per item for surface mail
   or $9.50 per item for airmail
** Washington State Residents add 8.4% Sales Tax

U.S Funds Only. Please allow 4-6 weeks for delivery. No C.O.D.

Sub total _____
*Shipping _____
** WA State Tax _____
Total _____

Name: _____
Address: _____
City: _____ State/Prov: _____
Country: _____ Zip Code: _____
Phone: _____ Fax: _____
Email: _____
Payment by: ❏ Visa   ❏ Mastercard   ❏ U.S. Check/International Money Order
Credit Card: # _____ Exp. Date: _____
Signature: _____

Order by:

Phone (360) 647-2703
Fax   (360) 647-0164
Email info@wellnesskinesiology.com

Please make check or money order payable to:
Topping International Institute Inc.
2505 Cedarwood Ave., Suite # 3
Bellingham, WA 98225

About the Author

DR. WAYNE TOPPING
–SPEAKER, EDUCATOR, AUTHOR

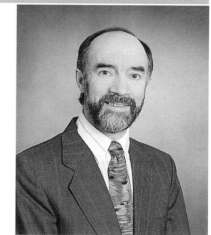

Wayne W. Topping, Ph.D., L.M.T., has a doctorate in geology from Victoria University in New Zealand, and was a geology professor with experience working on archaeology in the Middle East, active volcanoes in New Zealand, and glacial deposits in the Antarctic before he traded geology for an area he found even more fascinating – wholistic health.

While teaching geology in Southern California in 1976 Dr. Topping was introduced to Touch for Health. He expanded this interest in health by taking coursework in anatomy and physiology, nutrition, Swedish massage and other holistic courses.

By 1980 Wayne was ready to begin a new career in wholistic health. He trained at the Biokinesiology Institute in Talent, Oregon and become a certified Biokinesiology Instructor. He became a certified Massage Therapist in Washington State as well as an instructor in Touch for Health, and Educational Kinesiology.

Since 1984 he has written nine books, including: *Stress Release: Identifying and Releasing Stress Through the Use of Muscle Testing, Balancing the Body's Energies: Muscle Tests for the Eight Extra Meridians, Biokinesiology Workbook, What Makes You Tick is What Makes You Sick: Personality Traits and Their Relationship to Illness, Quake Busters: How to Defuse the Earthquakes in Your Mind,* and *Success Over Distress.* Most of his works have been translated into foreign languages. In addition to a busy writing and teaching schedule, Wayne is currently working on a doctorate in clinical hypnotherapy.

Dr. Topping has taught workshops in over 20 countries. He recently founded Wellness Kinesiology and has trained instructors who are currently teaching in Australia, Belgium, Brazil, Canada, England, France, Hungary, India, Italy, the Netherlands, Scotland, Southern Ireland, Switzerland, the United States and Zimbabwe.

If you are interested in information about books or seminars or would like to have Dr. Topping as a speaker or in-service trainer, please contact Topping International Institute Inc., 2505 Cedarwood Ave, Suite 3, Bellingham, WA, 98225 USA (360) 647-2703 Phone/Fax